HISTOLOGY AND EMBRYOLOGY

Mukhlisa Turopova

Histology and Embryology

by: Mukhlisa Turopova

Edition: December '2025

Publisher:

Taemeer Publications LLC (Michigan, USA / Hyderabad, India)

ISBN 978-93-6908-856-0

Book	:	**Histology and Embryology**
Author	:	Mukhlisa Turopova
Publisher	:	Taemeer Publications
Year	:	'2025
Pages	:	146
Title Design	:	*Taemeer Web Design*

SAFETY REQUIREMENTS AND RULES

A) general rules

Some of the heads and teachers of educational institutions biology instruments, devices, materials, as well as the source of energy that is used for the teaching of science in biology when dealing with damage to the health of the pupils must remember that constantly wrong.

The irresponsible, ignore the instrument is not familiar with the safety rules, do not know him, and as a result of not following undesirable phenomena can occur.

Such unpleasant events will not happen, so that each laboratory which demonstrated the process of transfer of experience and training to be considered a thorough safety by thinking from the viewpoint of the teacher, while the teacher's own experience should be an example in full compliance with safety rules.

The teacher to the students demonstrated experience unpleasant events that can happen before carrying out laboratory work and their prevention should give instruction on. The responsibility to follow the rules of safety will be the teacher who conducted the sessions with the students assume.

Consider doing so finds that those whom the same rule and biology teacher in the room hear the case and give information about safety rules that every reader will follow him special about the “safety of the notebook”ha must put their signature.

Science teachers in biology laboratory, laboratory head of the circle or not only, but also for their immediate guidance and full compliance with safety rules in the case of works by students on a regular basis must monitor.

Show students experience during training that are relevant to the excess of things that distract other styles of fantasy should not be on the table.

The heat balance equation for the temperature of the water in the learning process of 60-70 isitilayotgan^{0} S should not exceed.

Working of electrical equipment (elektroplitka, kavsharlagich electric, electric qaynatgich) you can't leave it unattended.

Buyers grass and quickly light the volatile fluid (air, gasoline, atseton, kerosene, alcohol and similar substances)alangalatib the risk of sending to them in the process of the experiment should stand away from the heater.

The use of gasoline as fuel, is absolutely forbidden.

In educational institutions of mercury used in laboratory work, show the transfer of experience is prohibited.

Security technical educational institution and school instruction written on the approval of the director of the laboratory room should be a place to hang put prominently visible.

B) Elis a welcome addition to safety rules

1. Before the use of electrical devices and the network it is necessary to become more familiar with their guidelines before connecting them to the network voltage corresponds to the voltage of the instrument intended that you should check. How they are all the part of the instrument to the surface of the vine, for the case of tension, poles and other information must be recorded.

2. All electrical tools(a microscope with an electric current running) from time to time in the prescribed manner of the condition and avoid that you need to examine a system or loamy.

Metal electrical devicesi's corps (the cover) should be connected to the ground of the world. It should be noted that the ground water connect-

pipes, the use of gas heater and is absolutely forbidden. Because the system of pipes and water heater radiators dielektrik (wood) and other insulated.

Electrical equipment, electrical measuring instruments and defects in wires connected to the suspect (if the special smell of smoke appears, and in other cases warms the wires) you need to immediately cut off the voltage. With the completion of work you need to disable electrical equipment immediately.

C) with the chemical safety of chemical agents used in the manufacturing process the rules of the technique

Some experience and a demonstrated experience in the provision of subject of biology, acid, salt, alkali in the water with the use of a solution comes on.Some of these substances may burn the point you need to remember to show the negative effects of poisons, and other supports. Such a situation not to happen it is necessary to observe the following safety rules:

1.Readers corrosive strong acid and alkaline solution, they work with is absolutely forbidden.

2. The smell of the ingredients in the detection of bending very close to the mouth of the container, steam or smell of gas coming out of a divorce can't. To do this, moving directly to the nose of engilgina kaft with steam or gas should be used with caution and take a breath. Depending on the flavor of the ingredients can not determine absolutely.

3. Study of biology-the laboratory of chemical agents in chemical manufacturing in the box is closed with a lock, network closet (seyf) and should be kept separated from other alkali

and acid manufacturing of chemical agents stored in biology as it is in the room.

4. Laboratory of chemical agents used in the room, which is closed with a stopper manufacturing all plastic, glass or ceramic containers should be stored in. The name of the substance and the concentration of the solution to the container, attached to the written paper must be put in. To toxic substances “Poison!”, easy burning a substance “to save from the grass!” the words must be put in writing.

5. You need to pour the acid into the acid solution in the preparation of the water. Ambitious to the container of acid and alkali solutionoyou need to slowly pour in using nk.

6. Chemical manufacturing chemical agents which have become unfit to work, to shed water rakovinasiga can't happen.

7. Touched to the skin or clothing of the person to acid, soda, nashatir with alcohol, acetic

acid alkali corrosive disinfection will be melted. Neytrallashtiruvchi substances must be booked in the room all the time.

The quality of the laboratory equipment requirements:

-due to scientific and technical progress of the present time lead;

-simple, comfortable, reliable be applied;

-aesthetic use the tool meets the requirements;

-safety rules gigienik give a complete answer to your requirements;

the laboratory equipment used in the experiment to show students be well visible;

-large size of all parts to be painted the color of the instrument;

-show the level of accuracy of the instrument used in the experiment, the responsiveness is great and high resistant to mechanical tension and robust;

-experience in spite of have the same results in repeated many times from far;

-the running time is not a necessity to set up or repair tools;

-scale and have demonstrated a clearly visible measuring instruments, which should stand them in a bright place or a digital tabloga.

1-LABORATORY LESSONS

WORK WITH THE MICROSCOPE. TEMPORARY AND PERMANENT DRUG PREPARATION

Lessonulot goali: the structure of the modern microscope and to learn the rules of working with it.

For training the necessary equipment: microscopes, slides and posters

The theoretical part of the training: optical microscope, if the item do the big shows are browsing a few times. At this time a combination of two of the optical system of the lens — system landscape — landscape okulyar primary system and directly shows that large — scale image shows the lens that gives: m: 8 times zoom lens with the zoom okulyar an image to show you the 7 must see and more, we investigates objects 56 times (7x8) zoom you will be browsing. It is noteworthy to say, seems to reverse the image in the microscope. If so, we have seen that the right side of the drug to the left, we have seen that the upper side, looking down we have moved. See the drug increases the size of the image in the microscope gently for a soft shift is recommended. Otherwise you want to see places from the area is going out.

Microscope mainly consists of 3 parts:

Access to all parts of the mechanical parts, while the force is the basis of the microscope (leg) and shtativ organizes. Shtativ — mechanical parts of the microscope, optical lens, combining lighting. The main part — it is in a solid condition taqasimon more leg and is convenient for installation. Shtativ different lenses in a different form, in the main function is to expose the revolver and the united comprehension is drastic. Tubusning okulyar in the upper part, while the object is located at the bottom. Prizmatik wallet is semi-spherical in shape, if the radical is secure with vint. In the research work which is used to track designed to get radical and binokulyar stereoskopik image with both eyes. Tubusni up and down for makrovint and mikrovintdan are used. Located in the lower part of tubusning Revolver, 3 or 4 slots behind , they object to the rotation of the revolver places and by various sized objects at a faster pace, there is the possibility of replacing. The mobility of the upper part of mikromexanizmning stolcha of items and sedentary places. Teach students stolcha on: go for the shake of the drug prujinasimon plastinkali ushlagichlar (zajim-klemma)—there are fiksatorlar. Stolcha items under a lighting device to mirror its structure and enter kondensor, they are the main part of the lighting apparatus. This light collected kondensor side members of the drug serves to stand up to the light.

Revolver and put the items that twists to the optical part of the microscope tubusga okulyar who put in the lobby. The weather'a welcome addition to the side in part I show them much larger than has been the number. Accordingly, the weather forecast'a welcome addition to weak, this isfar central and strong grassa strong bdieadi. Okulyar also weak (5.7), thiscentral peru (8x) and strong (15x) bdieib, the more indicated the same position is used.

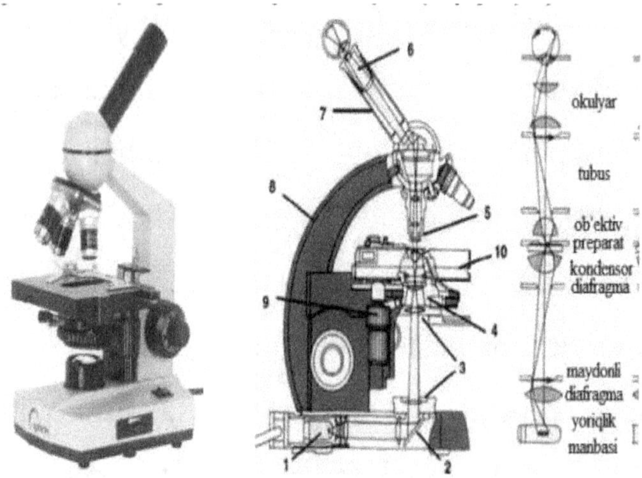

1-rasm. Mikroskop. Yorituvchi tizim: 1 – yorug'lik manbasi, 2 – oynacha, 3 – diafragma, 4 – kondensor; optik tizim: 5 – obyekt, 6 –okulyar; mexanik tizim: 7 – tubus, 8 – shtativ, 9 – kolonka, 10 – pridmet stolchasi

Thoroughly before working with a microscope, you need to get it installed. After that the mirror along the coast of the smallest set of lenses of the lens is put on the heavy side kondensor. Then you must complete the following:

1.Thoroughly installation of the microscope to the edge of the table, by placing a flat okulyar should be in the eye.

2.Find object by turning the mirror to focus light weak students to teach: a flat in the area of lighting you need. The mirror should be qamashtirmasligi light. 8x 40x digital (dry system) along the coast from the mirror when you are working with object heavy, 90x digital (fat) system is used while the lens when used with a flat mirror.

3.Items in stolcha the drug, the location of the object with the hole of the lens with stolcha to'g'risiga put klemmalar you need to secure.

4.Using makrovint focus is found.

5.Weak focus on objects at the desired level is observed and the drug is thoroughly secure.

6.The focus of the occurrences revolver when he turned the microscope, the lens weak object will be replaced. The revolver instead of the powerful object that fall chiqillashidan know you can.

7.The focus of using strong large original makrovint is found in caution, and are used to adjust mikrovintdan afford.

8.The drug has strong weather’a welcome addition to objective mikrovintning forward and back without interruption using to turn thisrga are. In a microscope, basically, is observed using the left eye, right eye, because the eye muscles must always be open without koordinatsiyalangan works. Shortened when the muscles of an eye, the latter of which also falls in the same situation. Initially interfere with the right eye like, later I will go to configure.

Adjuvant hardware after completion of the work using the picture are drawn. After that the drug product is taken from the lens is held stolcha and strong. When it breaks, because the drug does not get out from under a strong lens, the object can be broke. When working with a weak lens, kondensor is down, when used with strong, up is raised. This method uses the light and the convenient location of the drug is found in the details of what seems to be clear. The microscopic structures of the diaphragm of the microscope is a clear contrast ko'ringuncha should be closed.

Training to perform the procedure: 1. Shtativ microscope pile on the table to put the focus on yourself. Put small objects in the center of stolcha items on the strap. Okulyar the mirror and then left to see with the naked eye to the light source along the coast of the heavy side members follow that would be otherwise flat light.

2. So qo'yingki stolcha Perparat glass items of the object in the center or on the strap is verified okulyar stolcha. Then to'g'irlanadi the small lens using the focus range. To do this, the first product using a lens without an stolcha looking to mikrometr window qoplag'ich not to touch is to fall vint. Looking through okulyar then, turn slowly to the side and lift up tubusni

vintni mikrometr found yourself down. As a result, begin to be seen -- a glimpse of the object. Then edit vint mikrometr an interval more accurately focus the object ravshanlashtiriladi.

3. The great object of the microscope to monitor tubusni without the revolver twists, put the necessary items. Then, without looking down with an okulyar through clarification of the radical and the focus is mikrometr vint.

№	Girl and write digital microscope	
1		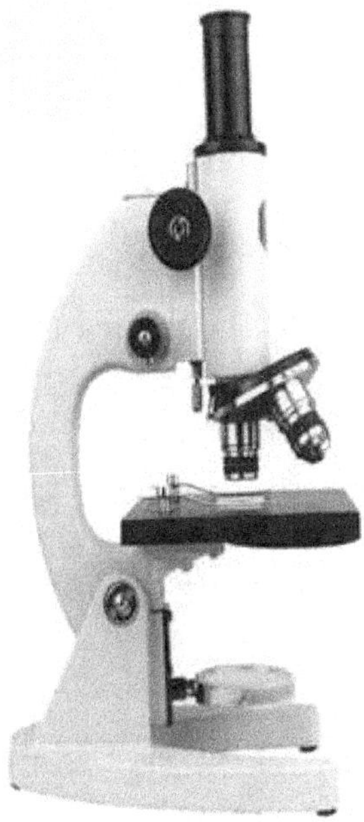
2		
3		
4		
5		
6		
7		
8		
9		
10		

The question of control

1. How the microscope parts?

2. The optical part of the microscope and its function what to include?

3. What to include and the part of the microscope illumination function?

4. What to include mechanical parts of the microscope and its function?

5. How to work with the microscope the rules of procedure?

6. Avzal modern microscopes and their line?

7. How you know the type of a microscope.

8. Phase contrast microscope and give information about interferensiya.

9. Polyarizatsion lyuminissent mikroskoplaryordamida and see what.

10. The working principles of the microscope and ultraviolet maydonli dark.

2-LABORATORY LESSONS CONSTANTLY PREPARATION OF THE DRUG

Job purpose: prepare and learn the technique of observation in the microscope prepat constant during practical sessions.

The necessary equipment for the job. microscopes, parts and qoplag'ich window, water dropper, petri dish, behind scalpel (onion skin, animal fur) visual of handouts.

Theoretical understanding. Sitora-histological inspections, typically, the biological term and permanent preparations from the object is prepared.

Permanent preparations of the preparation consists of several stages:

1) material; 2) to fiksatsiya; 3) wash; 4) suvsizlantirish - zichlashtirish; 5) to pour; 6)preparation of the incision; 7) painting; 8)the

incision suvsizlantirish; 9) lighting; 10) completion (the incision is closed with glass to yopqich). Get the material.

Progress of work: ***get the materials.*** In the case of small slices of the material to check it, murda during the dissection, the method is obtained by biopsy from living animals and people. The study drug for the preparation of animals mammals (dogs, cats, rabbits, rats) of the material obtained from the use of. To do this, send the air into the blood vessels (embolism) or slaughter (dekapitatsiya) slices of the drug from the body by way of the animals are killed and immediately take to prepare for that. When taking the study drug for the material, because it is necessary to give importance to his news a number of changes in the organs murda quickly that can happen. It is necessary to take material from murda within a period of 4-12 hours. The method of biopsy is often used for diagnostic purposes, therefore this method is used in experimental laboratories clinics and more.

Make Fiksatsiya. Fiksatsiya obtained it is necessary to make the material quickly. Fiksatsiya from the goal - is to maintain the structure of the vital tissue. Sitoplazma soak fiksatsiya defines the essence of protein cells. Thus, the protein will not be allowed to decay, as a result, the structure of cells and tissues is retained. Fiksatsiya conditions: a) the size of the piece 1-2 cm^3 should not exceed; b) bo'lakcha how small, will be so fiksatsiya quality; v) quality fiksatsiya fiksatorning size should be 100 times more than the size of which make fiksatsiya bo'lakcha; g) the term will be different depending on fiksatsiya fiksatorlarning kind. The painting method in which the drug implied fiksator likely the case that is selected. Almost all fiksatorlarning is used in some laboratories. Such fiksatorlarga include the following: a) 12% li formalin solution. To prepare

100% formalin 12 li^3 , get 88 cm^3 of water is added. Bo'lakcha taken to check the size of 1-2 cm^3 should not exceed. Doing so finds slices of whom 12% formalin for at least 24 hours from the purpose of the storage period ii fiksatsiya it also can hold a long time. You had to keep bo'lakcha years of formalin in the fluid, it is necessary to replace it every 3-4 months without liquid the stand. Then the tissue structure dramatically changes are not stored. The fine structure of the cells, functions in this way is not kept well. b) Myuller liquid/igi. 1 g of sodium and potassium for the preparation of the fluid myuller bixromat soo fat 2.5 g of salt, 100 cm^3 is dissolved in distilled water. 1 cm slices of $size^3$, it is desirable to be. Fiksatsiya lasts 7 days, it is necessary to replace it every day fiksatorni stand. Myuller fluid, usually, the amount is ready, it is prepared with a mixture of Formal Myuller at run time, that is, for every 100 cm^3 of fluid to 70 cm $Myuller^3$

formalin is added. This solution is used for the acceleration of tissue salts soak into xrom fiksatsiya because it slowly is going to fiksatsiya shortens the time while with the addition of formalin. The tissue was well preserved and later the general structure of such fluid paints different users. v) flemming's fluid. *Ingredients* 2%li xrom solution of 1% acetic acid acid consisting of li osmiy eritmasiva ice. The size of each tissue slices 1-2 cm^3. Fiksatorda days in a dark place they should stand for. *Advantages:* fine structure of the tissue was kept well only I will remain fiksatsiya not only that but also some tissue (fat, nerve fiber miyelinli) was painted black in color. g) jiksatori karni. Ingredients: 100° alcohol 12 cm $-^3$, -6 sm3 lantirilgan xloroform without water, ice acetic acid - 2sm3• This style is used for many gistokimyoviy fiksator. Whose slices 2-3 mm in $size^3$. Fiksatsiya muzxona time 1.5-2 hours. Thus, the fine structure and chemical composition of the cells is well kept. Quantitative gistokimyoviy tissues for conducting inspections and fs fiksatori is widely used in recent times. Ingredients: 100% li 60 cm^3 formalin, with 1000 20 cm^3 6 cm alcohol and^3 consisting of acetic acid is. Organoid cells to determine the max fiksatorlar sus available: mitoxondriya for - Reg fiksatori, Golji fiksatori for complex aoyama and others. As noted above, this depends on the goal that put fiksatorning before he or researcher to be applied.

Wash. After completion of fiksator is fiksatsiya pour the slices are washed in water. After some fiksatorlardan (alcohol, karni, the shabada liquid, and others) in the next stage directly without washing the tissue - to suvsizlantirish is held.

Suvsizlantirish- zichlantirish. After washing, the slices in the heat of an increased spirtlar 50° starting from, 60°, 70°, 80°, 90°, 96° finally 100°, i.e. in absolute spirtlar zichlashtiriladi. Spirtlar suvsizlanish and was zichlash in slices.

Transplant. Spirtlar slices in ma'ium had zichlashib level, despite the fact that it's hard to get a still thin enough bo'imaydi incision, therefore the next stage is integrated with a special substance in them. Then only play the role of density slices xii them the opportunity to cut a thin incision is born. You should learn tissue: selliodin, wax, selloidin-wax and gelatin, take a look. Electronic microscopic inspections or after the animal has been killed at the time of biopsy tissue slices for 1 to 2 minutes must include fiksatorga look. Only then can the fine structure of the cells and organoid them well preserved. Fiksatorlar osmiy acid mainly as 1-4% solution glutaraldegidning li and 3-6%solution of li is used. Fiksatsiya osmiy process in acid solution for 1.5-2 hours, lasts from 6 hours to several days glutaraldegidda. Fiksatsiya after increasing the concentration of the slices in the spirtlar suvsizlantirilib metakrilat, anabol, aral, vestopal synthetic smolalar seems to look like.

To cut. Made from a special steel blade slices and laid to wax selloidin chana mikrotomda of using cut. It is desirable to be 7-8-10 mk qaliniigi selloidin of incision. The thickness of the incision 5-7 wax mk. The chana mikrotomlardan in addition, muzlatuvchi mikrotomlar are also available, such mikrotomlarda only new or fiksatsiya made, but is cut slices singdirilmagan zichlantirilmagan wax and other substances. Using slices of frozen carbon dioxide in hard condition. Which put them in the preparation of synthetic drugs for electronic mikroskopiya smolalar slices max rnikrotomlar sus - ultramikrotomlarda diamond or glass using a knife made from a very thin incision when they specifically seem to look the net. This incision thickness of 200 to 300 A (angstrem)1, if it is 200-300 times the wax from the incision is thin.

Painting. XiI index of the structural elements of the cells colorless and absorption of the light reason, it is necessary to see them painted. The components of the cell it should be painted with various paints to see them because they have different chemical properties. Thus, dyes and paints with sour sitoplazma features which have alkaline properties hujayralararo substance of the cell, while the core was painted. rem angst (A)-D,OOO mk. The core of most supported paints: 1. Gemotoksilin qarnish tayyorlanuvchi tree plant oil paint is a color that was painted purple to the core. 2. See also: deaf - animal oil painting, was painted a red color to the core. 3. Alkaline - anilin dyes (gensian - violet krezil - violet, methyl-violet, ishqori - fuksin and others). The most supported and cons paint a pink color from cells eozin sitoplazrnasini hujayralararo substance were painted, painted a red color while the same structures was sent. In addition, there are special paints for certain components of tissues and cells: 1) sudan III, sudan black fats, the fat cells and nerve fibers were painted red or black color; 2) paint two walls for the painting of elastic fibers rnavjud - orsein - a liver and was painted the dark color of elastic fibers rezorsin - fuksin of elastic fibers were painted in a pink color; 3) to determine the tissue fibers and nerves are painted with silver nitrate salt argirofil them. Paint one where they are used, a simple painting, two or more when used in paints, for example, and sour-based paint when applied at the same time, the complex is called a painting. The painting method most frequently used to enter the following complex: 1) gematoksilin-painted with eozin. This method to know the structure of paint is applied as a general organ or tissue.

Painting procedure: incision gematoksilinga is put in 5-10 minutes, and then rinsing in water for about 2-3 minutes eozinga shall be re-rinsing in water, and then only suvsizlantiriladi, the lighting, and the end is passed. The color purple drug core, sitoplazma hujayralararo are painted in pink color and substance; 2) upon your business Van method: this method allows a better view of muscle tissue and collagen fibers. The drug in the cells of the core to'qjigar color, sitoplazma sariqqa hungry, dark sariqqa, connective tissue are painted a red color; 3) the method is applied for Veygert elastic fibers. 4) are the two major fiber or painted on argirofil gomori method; 5) methods for the detection of nerve tissue with silver nitrate is applied to the salt impregnatsiya-Bilshovskiy to the central nervous system, peripheral nervous system Gross-Bilshovskiy method are used. Identify and briefly the structure of the chemical substances in tissues and cells number and their location which allows you to track gistokimyoviy painting methods are also available. For example, the best method to determine polisaxaridlar, we have rollers - reaction method to detect RNA Brashe, the dna method to determine Fyolgen and others. While electronic microscopic preparations are painted with heavy metal salts and salt uranilatsetat qo'rg'oshinning sitrat. Suvsizlantirish the incision. After painting spirtda suvsizlantiriladi of the incision.

Lighting. After the incision of the rays of light or a crisp suvsizlantirilgandan be very good for lighting needed them to be. The following is the substance lighting: I. Carbon - xylene 2. 3 xylene or toluene. Chinnigul oil and others. In the article the coverage of the incision 0.5 - minutes I hold it.

Completion. To summarize, canada or balzak kedr is used. The incision despite it biriktiribgina remain, but the coverage of the drug also helps. The glass was attached to the subject detached from the substance covering the incision, and it instilled 1 drop balzak yopqich with window are closed. Then only it will be ready to see. Drug and examined using a light microscope, are studied. Remove them from-I type is most often applied in the practical works of the microscope, microscopes for different special research in polyarizatsion, phase contrast, the use of microscopes and other ultraviolet light. In addition, the students teach: object zoom microscope has wide application in the electronic proud provider of scientific research. Microscope structure, work process and all use given in textbooks and manuals.

The question of control

1. What are the stages of how to prepare prepat permanent?
2. What is the purpose of making fiksatsiya?

3. Ready to provide permanent prepat what is the purpose?

4. Avzal modern microscopes and their line?

5. How you know the type of a microscope.

6. Phase contrast microscope and give information about interferensiya.

7. Polyarizatsion lyuminissent mikroskoplaryordamida and see what.

18. The working principles of the microscope and ultraviolet maydonli dark.

3-LABORATORY LESSONS
THE STRUCTURE OF BIOLOGICAL MEMBRANES AND PLAZMOLEMMA

Training goali: plazmolemma during laboratory sessions and study the structure of biological membranes.

Kvery era equipment: microscopes, visual handouts, drugs prepared.

Theoretical understanding

Sitoplazma of all body cells and tissues from the external environment the third floor - floor - foreign distinguishes shell. Thus, sitolemma or plazmolemma is also called ... The average thickness of 7.5 nm is equal to his, are not seen in the light microscope. Accordingly, the microscope is used to study its structure only. The shell is composed of two chetki oqsildan the floor, the middle floor consists of yog'simon substance. Tiny membrane in the strap if you want to pass through them into the cells of the substances, substances out of waste that is generated as a result of the exchange of substances. Pinositoz and different in structure and membrane properties of dissolved substances fagositoz particles of liquid drops surrounded sends the ice. Consequently, the physiological function of the outer membrane of the cell to the cells of the necessary nutrients, unnecessary, out of the ice, is to ensure the integrity of the cell activities of life and stand out. The outside and the inside of the membrane sprouting o'simtasi people will be there. These o'simtasi as they formed with the layer directly attaching to adjacent cells, that depends on the interaction with them, that will ensure a solid and communication. Inside the inner product on the hand out of the floor, and just go until sitoplazma the core part with, but will react with the core. Of the function. The internal environment of the cell from the external viscosity, chemical composition, structure, ion and many other physical and chemical properties, according to tevarak - the environment is different. The outer membrane of the cell from the external environment and the internal environment was kept for the entire life of this difference is limited. This hole ions through the membrane into the cells, tiny molecules of water and other substances, for example, glucose will take. Accessing external to the cell membrane of ions and molecules from the external environment that would regulate it out to you. Molecules and ions, i.e. with constant exchange of various substances between cells occur in the external environment such stands.

The progress of the work: prepared for students of the membrane structure and structure originally plazmolemma through colorful pictures will become familiar with the components. Then through a microscope to see the structure of the prepared drug in plazmolemma are studied. It also plazmolemmaning the structure and composition of the image seen in the microscope and draw students attention is given to the album.

Control questions and assignments

1. Tell Plazmolemmaning functions
2. What is the structure consists of structural Plazmolemmaning
3. Let me explain protein and lipid Plazmolemmadagi your footprint.
4. The structure of biological membranes've drawn the picture

4-LABORATORY LESSONS
SITOPLAZMA OF ORGANOID - ENDOPLAZMATIK LACE, RIBOSOMA, GOLJI STRUCTURE OF APPARATUS

Hobbiesto order: Endoplazmatik lace, peroksisoma, sferasomalar, Golji study the structure and function of the apparatus.

The necessary equipment for training: computer technology, proektor, posters and slides

Lessonulot of content: Endoplazmatik netoil and gas are two different types of:

1) Granulyar or atg'al

2) smooth endoplazmatik nets.

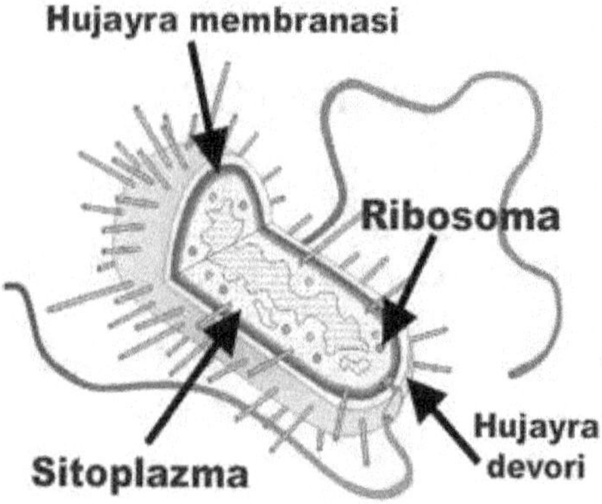

Endoplazmatik mesh of the membrane chemical compositionwere determined by biochemical analysis I. In its structure there are proteins and lipids. Besides, how much an enzyme, for example, ATP – azaga have

This organoid are found in all plant and animal cells, but bacteria areas lyddaqit is not clear stained.

Granulyar endoplazmatik

4.1-picture. The basic structure of the cell

tthisrning sintezida protein was clear proof of participation. Smooth endoplazmatik tthisfor the synthesis of glycogen and lipid in the membrane r identified.

Net endoplazmatik both in the same channel, and vakuollarida sisterproduct of the synthesis of proteins in the world, eitherg's and t of glycogenthisis plab.

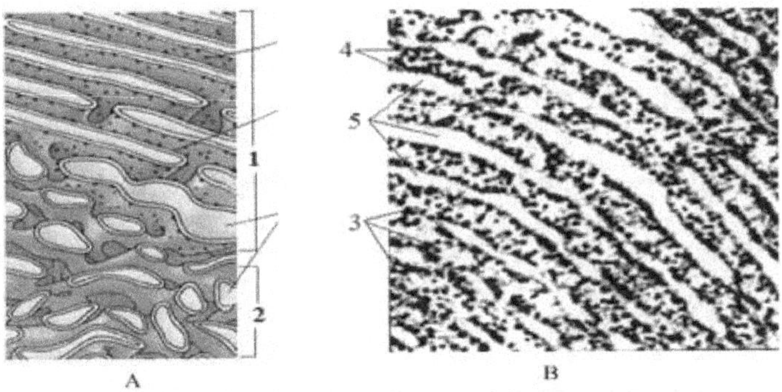

12-rasm. A –Endoplazmatik to'r (sxema). B –Donador endoplazmatik to'rning elektron mikroskopda ko'rinishi: 1–donador endoplazmatik to'r; 2– silliq endoplazmatik to'r; 3–ribsssmalar, 4–membrana; 4–endoplazmatik to'r bo'shlig'i.

Until the present time net endoplazmatikng qcannot be formed from the material to determine was working. However, this is so foreign that is in contact with the membrane yakindan sitoplazmatik organoid or at the expense of those being in contact with the membrane at the expense of his core yakindan endoplazmatik tthisr of the membrane can be formed projections should be. The following analysis confirmed this assumption. Microscopic examination of wheat endosperm cells in its computer's electronic haltasimon will be to identify the eaves of the nuclear membrane form the net of it while endoplazmatik sisters is formed.

Qistheacha reviews

- Are bound to one tube, and cystic qopcha network.

Funkyalar will:

- sitoplazmathe top layer of his qalinlashtiradi lekarzem.
- sitoplazmaensures internal stability of muslims under.

➢ the metabolicproduct of k in the synthesis ofi, and stored to moveiat participating.

➢ the synthesis of steroids and proteins in cells, glycogen and performs functions such as storage and to ensure the placing of membrane protein.

Ribosoma the net incoming endoplazmatik content, circular in shape, the diameter is equal to 150-350 is a structure, they only can be seen in the electronic microscope. In the cell, usually two xii ribosoma if endoplazmatik net many of them structured in the membrane part, the second part or in sitoplazma free without mitoxondriya or xloroplast matriksida also occurs. Some time to be had with them in which rna axboriy, ulargapoliribosomalar is called. Ribosoma 40% of I k rn 60% consists of protein. Two subbirlikdan is Ribosoma. Then the ir or mr k k, which form a chain which had polipeptid place and tRNK-c available.

Functions. Ribosoma the function of protein synthesis. In the cell, consequently, in the structure of all the proteins is synthesized in the organism ribosoma. Sitoplazma aminokislota of protein molecules in each cell in ribosoma from the assembly. Proteins, basically, is synthesized in the membrane of net accumulated in structured endoplazmatik ribosoma. Protein synthesis complex --

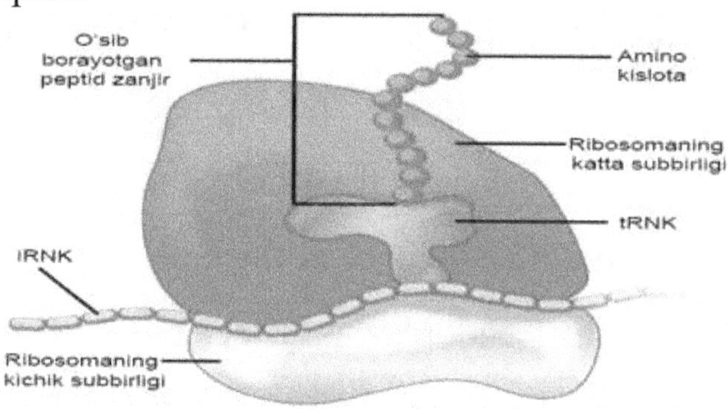

4.3-picture. Ribosoma structure.

the process is not only ribosoma, but how much of the package is carried out through a dozen ribosoma. Ribosoma poliribosoma of such a collection is called. The proteins synthesized initially structured endoplazmatik channel and transported to the cavity of the net, it is they consume. Ribosoma of proteins and carrier who is the only biosintezi Endoplazmatik and net hardware.

Golji apparatus. Available in two different hardware Golji the condition of family structure: consists of separate structures and plant cells that are specific to to'rsimon - diffuse form. Made from will determine the three golji using electronic microscope is identical to the hardware:

1. Sis is smooth and wrapped with a membrane located near the core consists of sisternalar. They fosforlanish proteins in transit, will take to be medial. Sister's area is updated regularly here. They endoplazmatik mesh is formed from smooth.

2.Medial is located in the transit consists of three sister if tiny bubbles will take to be undergone changes of the protein in trans.

3.Is Trans - located in the central part of the implementation of vakuol distended sisternalar of them consist plazmatik is located close to the membrane.

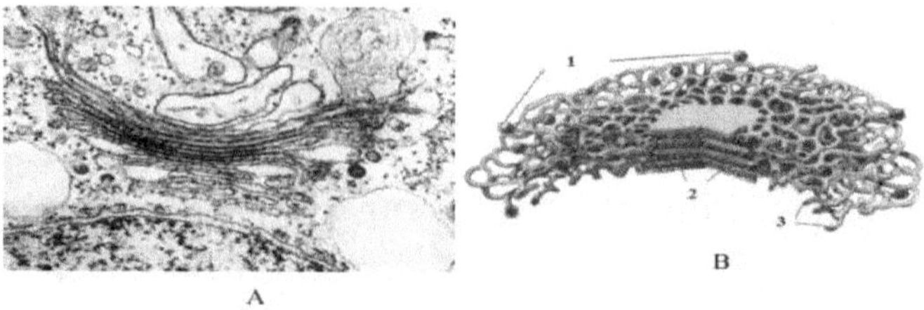

14-rasm. Golji kompleksining elektron mikroskopda ko'rinishi (A) va ultramikroskopik tuzilishi (sxema) (B): 1- pufakcha; 2- membrana bilan o'ralgan yassi sisternalar; 3- naychalar.

Golji in hardware are two separate zones: proximal and distal.

The proximal part of the process of growing cells and the nucleus in different sekret sitoplazma, the distal portion is facing to the outside of the cell.

Qi proximalcmpufakchali tinyr sisternalar settles and short, this place is the place to golji endoplazmatik net hardware. If it reaches the distal portion having a large vakuol, sekresiya filled with product inside of them.

Golji the functions of the apparatus. The bubbles collect in the synthesized product net hardware golji endoplazmatik of membranes, is involved in chemical change and reaching. Apparatus Golji sisterin the world and the synthesis of products with hardware and most importantly the night polisaxaridlar mukoproteidlar golji sekret is excreted out of the cells.

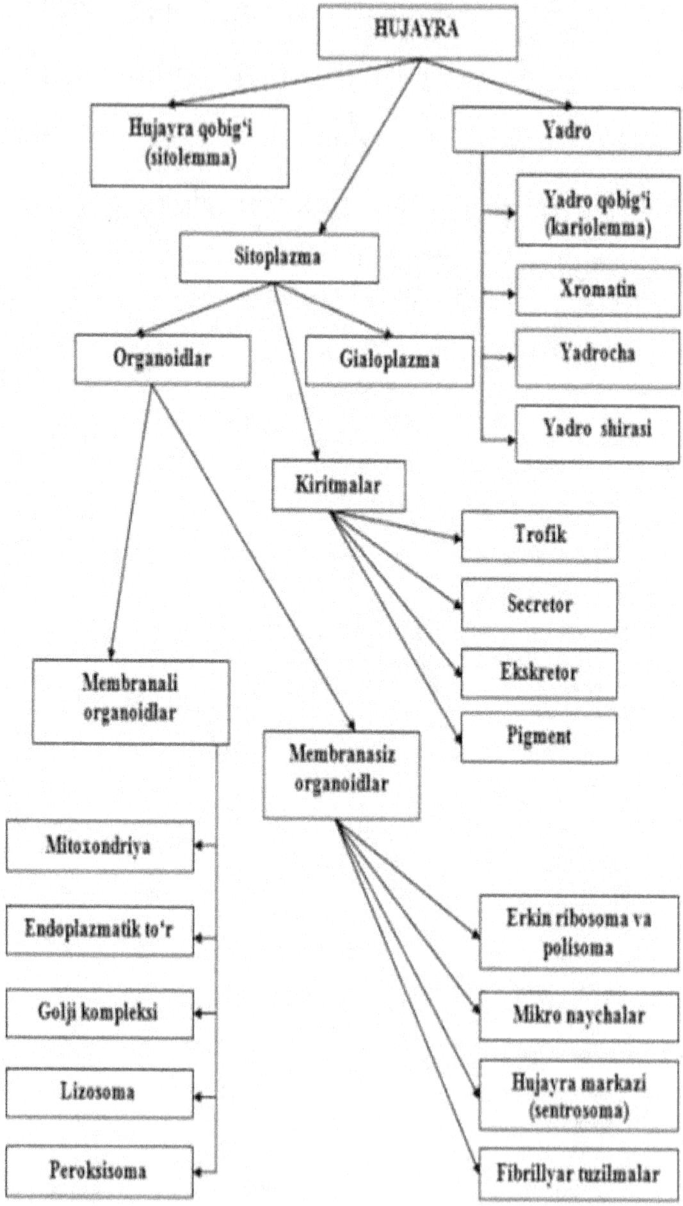
HUJAYRA
Hujayra qobig'i (sitolemma)
Yadro
Yadro qobig'i (kariolemma)
Xromatin
Yadrocha
Yadro shirasi
Sitoplazma
Organoidlar
Gialoplazma
Kiritmalar
Trofik
Secretor
Ekskretor
Pigment
Membranali organoidlar
Membranasiz organoidlar
Mitoxondriya
Endoplazmatik to'r
Golji kompleksi
Lizosoma
Peroksisoma
Erkin ribosoma va polisoma
Mikro naychalar
Hujayra markazi (sentrosoma)
Fibrillyar tuzilmalar

Endoplazmatik net net is collected and synthesized in protein export apparatus in ribosoma endoplazmatik sisternalar golji is transported to the zone of the membrane. Here endoplazmatik net protein filled tiny vakuol are separated, the proximal part of the apparatus Golji vakuol enter into the zone. Vakuol here are collected and sisternalar is added with each other and in the same manner. Protein granules or liquid collected after that to become sekretor can be left without. Then Golji apparatus and sisterare separated from each other s will join with oqsilli vakuol yiriklashib. This membrane with the membrane of the membrane plazmatik vakuol are added and they can move towards plazmatik in vakuollar of the inside of the product is excreted from the cell. Pinotsitozga ekzotsitozdir reverse this process. Endoplazmatik net export proteins synthesized in a structured, for example, digestive enzymes from the cell to the outside of the apparatus passive Golji case (proferment) out of the water. Funksat iona reached the placeigo become, this proferment becomes active. For example, thrips enzymes in the duodenum becomes active. Oxirgacha studied the mechanisms of this process, but it is necessary to go to their atp. Golji in hardware as well as metabolic process, go to the modification of proteins occurs.

Brief description:

• IwhoiyaKamilla Golji social biology dedicated to the name ofsistercalled about a s many of vakuol theworld was founded. In the cells of plants diktiosomis called many years ago.

Funkyalari:

• Endoplazmatik proteins and lipids, which is formed retikulumda stores, packaging, and distribution.

• Proteins designed for himself and make a difference at the "traits" having the character of proteins recognizes and back, endoplazmatik retikulumga sends.

- Cell sitokinezduring cell platethe shape of the asi.
- Some carbohydrates to protein synthesis binds to the cell membrane and makes polisaxaridlar.

The progress of the work: Students endoplazmatik lace, the structure of hardware and golji ribosoma ready with color photos, pictures of finished drugs in the form of permanent or electro through the video, are introduced. Draw pictures of drug seen through a microscope constant after that. Thus, net, net, and structured to focus on e'tibir endoplazmatik ribosoma endoplazmatik empty. The bubbles and permanent preparatda golji sisternalar don't find in hardware. Carefully pay attention to the composition of ribosoma.

The question of control

1. Golji hardware is sis
2. Golji hardware is medial
3. Golji of the apparatus is trans
4. The functions of the apparatus Golji
5. Hardware key in the metabolism of substances in the cells of Golji “full setups available” explain the role as organoid.
6. Let us explain the structure of net Endoplazmatik

5-LABORATORY LESSONS SITOPLAZMA OF ORGANOID - LIZOSOMALAR, SENTRASOMA, THE STRUCTURE OF MIKRONAYCHALAR

Hobbiesto order: lizosomalar, sentrasoma, mikronaychalar of the structure and function study.

The necessary equipment for training: computer technology, proektor, posters and slides

Lessonulot of content: Lizosomalar- Brief sherh

- Cells in organoidthe major structure of the world, it is very necessary for the cells. In all koldiqlarni and outdated organoidwhich s digest enzymesare there. Lizosomalar cells will digest quickly after you kill them. Lizosomalar would have remained dead skin cells without living cells.

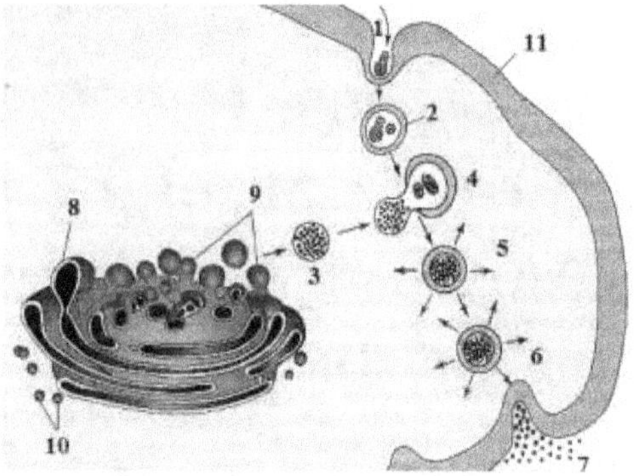

15-rasm. Hujayra ichida modda parchalanishiniig ultramikroskopik sxemasi: 1–fagotsitozlanuvchi tana; 2–hazm vakuolasi; 3 – birlamchi lizosoma; 4– endotsitoz; 5,6–ikkilamchi lizosoma; 7–tashqariga chiqarilgan tanachalar; 8–Golji apparat sisternalari; 9–Golji apparati vakuollari; 10- mikropufakchalar; 11- hujayra membranasi.

Functions:

- the cells will help the erosion of large molecules
- provides protection from bacteria and viruses
- in the time of famine they themselves will digest them showing the effects on personal organoid cells

- leads to the death of these cells.

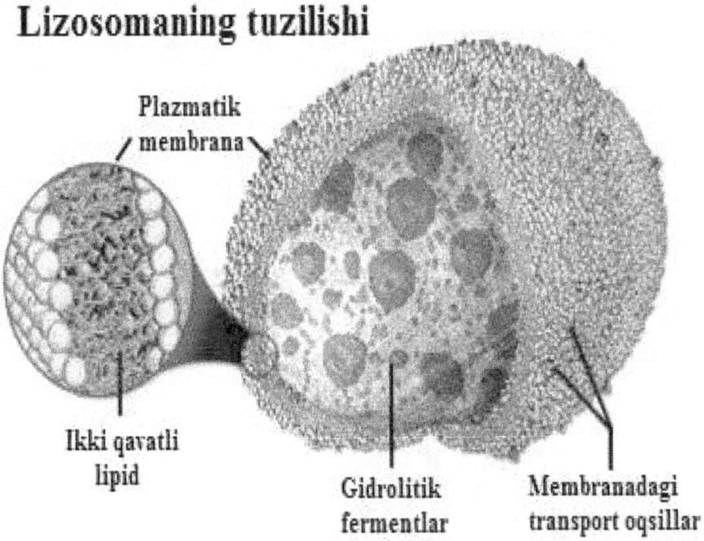

Therefore they are called lizosomalar bags which you can kill.

Peroksisoma - eukariot organoid cells is universal. Like Lizosomalar K.De found by Dyuv. The floor is wrapped with a membrane, the membrane is a fluid mosaic structure. Kristallsimon in structure - nukleoidi is (no connection to the core). He and fibrill

5.2-picture. Take lizosomalar structure.

mikronaychalar is uratoksidaza enzymes, lizosomalardan only be increased by different peroksisomaning available. Therefore, the cells can't restore lost peroksisomalarini own them. Biochemical oxidation reactions in the enzymes of them Peroksisomalarning function (katalaza), which is associated with the substances to be formed as a result of the breakdown of hydrogen peroxide-(cells) will decompose to water and oxygen. Hydrogen peroxide is formed as a result of the reactions in the cells that go very harmful and toxic to the cell must be out. Enzymes decompose to water and oxygen content in fulfilling this task peroksisomalar katalaza it.

Umumhujayraviy function with the composition of long chain fatty acids from the breakdown of nutrients to the cells in. Alcohol liver cells of the body to be rich peroksisomalarga falling 30%i in here acetatealdegid and acetic acid to decomposenordi. Alcohol (English- *al~kuhl-fine* powder) and long-term low doses isle'mol to increase the amount of acetic acid in the structure of liver cells and lead to the establishment of the synthesis of more fatty acids. As a result, increased the amount of lipid sirrozi (Greek-yellow) develops the disease.3 peroksisomalar occurring in plants, make up the group:

1. Glioksisomalar-used to decompose the oil-rich seeds of lipids in saxaroza will participate.

2.Peroksisomalar mitoxondriya occurring in the leaves and is involved in breathing associated with plastida.

3. Differensiatsiyalanmagan peroksisomalar occurring in other tissue types.

The center of the cell, i.e. sentrosoma. All animals and plants found in the cells of tubal organelladir Sentriol. For the first time, Flemming F. (1875) is determined. The first time it is found in cells bo'linayotgan sentrosoma at the time. Later inspections as a result of ma'lum neckldick, sentrosoma bo'linayotgan cells compared to other cells see the good in it. This is removed in the form of two simple organella sentriola to afford a light microscope. In the microscope, such as electronic, that is not cylindrical sentriola tanacha length 0,3-0,5 mkm in diameter and 0.1 - 0,15 mkm. Its walls consist of thin pair 9 naysimon collection. Each package is located in the tube than 3, if the triple is called. Sentriolaning length is equal to the length of each triple. Sentriolalar pair-a pair are placed perpendicular to each other. Sentriola axis defines the axis to be. Sferik Sentriolalar settles in the center of mass in this mass *, or sentroplazma sentrofera* is called. Sentroferada membrane is not according to the density, rich in protein and sitoplazma is quite different.

The internal structure or composition that

have been xivchini kiprikchalar sentriolaning in some sources is similar. Check electronic microscope was carried out in a truly confirms the presence of similarities between them.

Basal cells are cylindrical in shape, like mikronaychalar sentriola 9 pairs, consists of. This time the task of the cell until sentriolaning be tied to come. Xivchini is formed on the present data and the network that is involved in sentriolalar lashes have found.

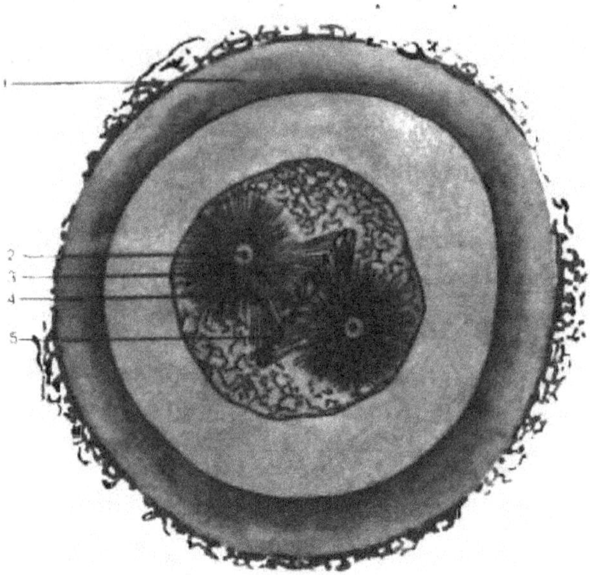

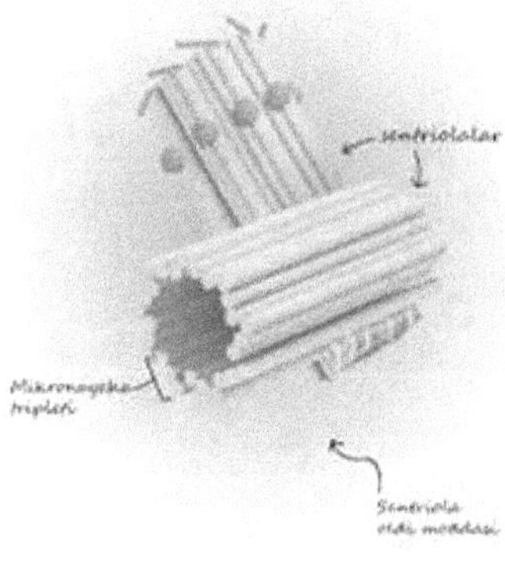

5.3-picture. ***Bo'linayotgan x 900 sentrosoma in the egg cell.***

1-egg po 'stlog 'i; 2-sentriolalar; 3-sentrosfera;

4-astrosfera; 5-chromosome is located in the equator.

Also located in the same mikronaychalar sitoplazma sentriola and basal cells, consists of. They usually performs the function of the base form and the setting. Mikronaychalar obtained from the chemical structure of the cells of most animals is almost the same, basically, I find oqsildan specific tubulin content.

The progress of the work: lizosomalar Students during lessons, and the structure sentrasoma mikronaychalar ready with color photos, presentations or carp are seen in a microscope and the image to read through a constant drug they can.

Control questions and assignments

1. Lizosomalar've functionality.
2. Peroksisomalarning in the cell what is the function consists of.
3. Stell entrasomolarning structure and function.
4. Thematic've drawn images.

6-LABORATORY LESSONS

SITOPLAZMA OF ORGANOID - PLASTIDA AND THE STRUCTURE OF MITOXONDRIYA

Hobbiesto order: plastida of Mitoxondriya and study the structure and function.

The necessary equipment for training: computer technology, proektor, posters and slides, prepared drugs.

Lessonulot of content: mitoxondriya organellalar regulating the synthesis of atp, the cell's energy system builds. Sitoplazma in donasimon, ipsimon structures called mitoxondriya (mitoz — ip chondros — pieces). The electronic structures of four's mainly by mitochondria under the microscope seems to be clear: outer membrane, inner membrane, crystals, and matri perks. Mitoxondriya mkm thickness of 0.5 in length can be up to 1 to 10 mkm Mkm. It gialoplazmadan mitoxondriya of the outer membrane, inner membrane, while it distinguishes matriksidan.

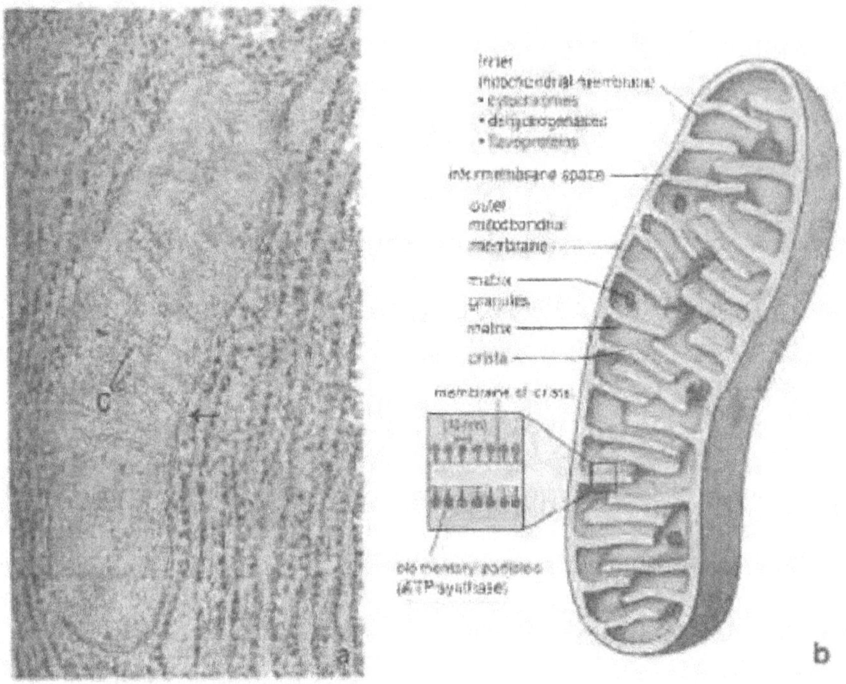

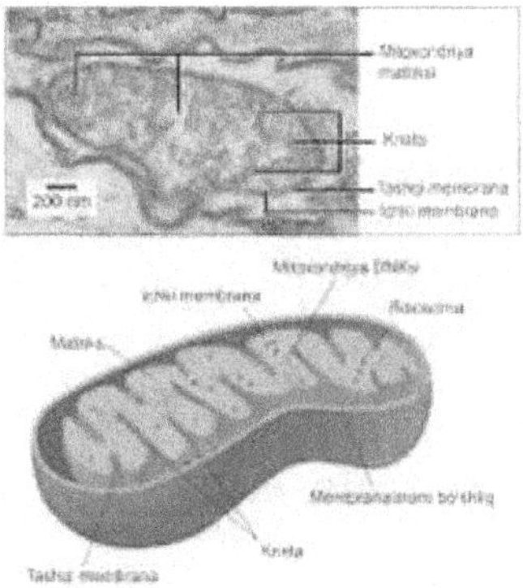

6.1-picture. Mitoxondriya and their structure.

A —v — mitoxondriya knew plastinkasimon crystals:

A — scheme; V - TEM; C—D - pufaksimon knew mitoxondriya crystals; S - scheme; D - TEM: 1 - outer membrane; 2 — the gap between the membrane; 3 — inner membrane;

4 — the crystals; 5 — matri perks.

Two membrane o ‘rtasi cavity in the inner membrane into the overhang of perks from matri — crystals are bulging out of. Crystals in the face of tiny round particles, the particles are fermented in regulating the synthesis of atp this. Mitoxondriya matri, tamoxifen er can be. Mitoxondriya the average life span of 10 days. To allocate a certain portion out of the way they split or increased. Mitoxondriya their DNKsi, have to ribosoma. The kidney is involved in steroid hormone gland usi mitoxondriya sintezida, while the crystals will be in the form of tiny bubbles. (6.1-picture).

They specifically xloroplast specific to the green pigment in green color - depends on the existence at xlorofil. Xloroplast and other green leaf of the plant in the cells of the body. Green plants use energy from xlorofil to be the light of the sun could synthesize organic compounds from inorganic substances and takes his account. Organic substances from inorganic substances, ya 'the process of being formed to carbohydrates is called photosynthesis. Xloroplast often oval-shaped, 4-6mkm is sized. High plant 40-60 xloroplast usually occurs in a single cell. Xloroplast electronic structure of thin was detected using a microscope. Sitoplazma xloroplast about 40000 times when you zoom in, from a two - outer and inner membrane is limited because it looks good. Outer and inner membrane, the outer membrane of the cell mitoxondriya also structured as three from the floor. Inside Xloroplast semi-liquid substance that fills, then just separate structures specific to xloroplast - the facets are in. The facets in the form of a cylindrical membrane formed from flat located one on top of each other the first jesuit bag. This bag by area dm stack-column stack level of the coins is going to like; the structure up to 50 facets in one-a bag of such area may be. The rounded edges of ko'ndalangiga qirqim seems to be. A few facets are xloroplast one in ten. All facets of the interaction with the membrane of xloroplast combined. Xloroplast various plant-sitoplazma the part of the cell in the heart: the flower, the fruit, the stem, the leaves in. Xloroplast a different form of many small crystals or 5-6 in length, and they often come mkm girrali that has the characteristics of the needle. Various autumn leaves and fruits of each district xiI Gultojibarglar sarig, zarg'aldog and keep your business depends on xloroplast fail to be in color. Leykoplastlar colorless. They are colorless sitoplazma the parts of the plant, for example, in the stem, roots and tubers is removed to afford. Leykoplastlarning every form xiI. Often these long-term has the form of rounded or tayoqcha mkm 5-6. Potato starch grains leykoplastlarga who gather tugunak common example. Xloroplast the xromoplastlar leykositlar and can become mutually to each other. Photosynthesis use energy from the sun is the synthesis of organic compounds, inorganic substances, this process was plastida in the night.

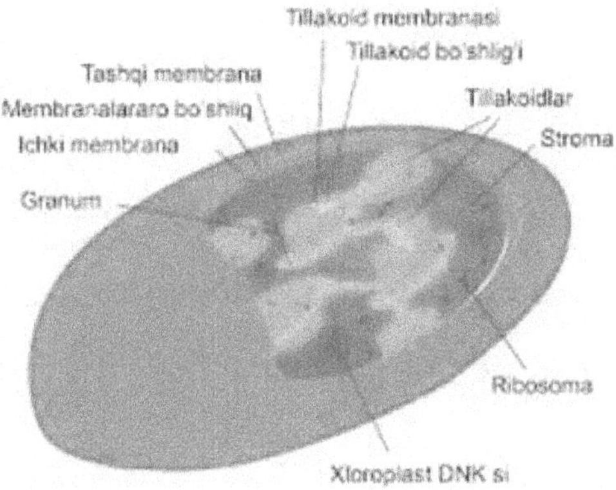

The light phase. As a result, the water translates into energy to light energy fotolizi ximik. As a result, atp and NADF.N is formed. This process tilakoidlarda night.

6.2-picture. Plastida structure.

The phase of darkness: this process stromalarda night. Atp is synthesized as a result of this process and reactions of organic compounds and the number NADF.The presence of N appears. Glucose is stored in the position or falls to yield polymeric sitoplazma.

Out of work: the theoretical part of the lesson students acquainted with medicines prepared after chiqqanlaridan, color pictures, or through video presentations and mitoxondriya will learn the structure of plastida. Thus, the internal mitoxondriya composition, means of appropriate agreements in which the crystals of the matri perks and pay attention. Carefully follow the structure of plastida. Tilakoidlar means of appropriate agreements and give importance to the strong part. Ava plastida mitoxondriya structure on a sheet, learn drawing the top picture.

Control questions and assignments

1. How mitoxondriya structured?
2. Mitoxondriya of function?
3. That's basically it seems clear multiple electronic structures under the microscope by mitochondria?
4. A few of the membrane wrapped with xloroplast floor?
5. Where is the phase of light kich?

6. Plastida glucose, which is formed in a part of?
7. Take a picture and the organoid structure of organoid get acquainted with drew.

7-LABORATORY LESSONS

ENTER CELL

Lesson aim: to study the structure and function of the cells.

The necessary equipment for training: computer technology, proektor, color photographs, and slides.

Training content: sitoplazma cells associated metobolizmga It is going to be lost, can appear to be. It trophic, sekretor, and pigment types ekskretor.

In the cells *of trophic it* occurs a lot, they are proteins, carbohydrates, fats will be in the form of. It is simple and in the case of complex proteins protein. In some proteins, carbohydrates, fats, with or without lipoproteidlar which had, in the form of a lot glikoproteidlar occurs. Often glycogen carbohydrates (e.g., liver cells) will be in the form of. Circular in the form of fat, in a large variety of it is in the process of synthesis is formed.

Ekskretor enter, the cell will be sent out as special and sintezlanmaydi metabolite.

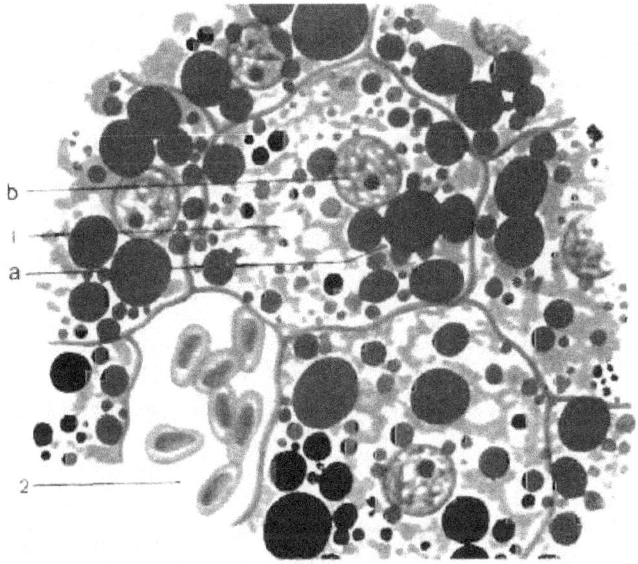

Pigment enter, the endogenous and exogenous to endogenous melanie, miozin, hemoglobin, and bilirubin in the lobby. Enter a pigment, pigment cells occurs and is synthesized in a special lot. It comes importation of exogenous pigment.

Sekretor enter, and, basically, gland cells, they are circular, **7.1-picture. Fat droplets in the liver cells.**

1-inflammation of the liver;

a-a drop of fat; b-core; 2-eritrotsit with kapil.

ekzokrinositlarda sitoplazmnsida apical cells, all cells on the side of endokrinositlarda sitoplazma occurs.

The progress of the work: read the theoretical part of the training, then enter it in the cells of the liver and permanent preparatda in the picture, pay attention to the type and the composition.

Control questions and assignments

1. How it is different from the organoid?
2. How it is to be in the group?
3. What are the cells of the gland was it?
4. Enter bilirubin, which is an example of the type?

8- LABORATORY LESSONS

NUCLEAR STRUCTURE

Lesson aim: students and its core components, the core and the external apparatus, give understanding about the role in the activity of the core cell life. Give students understanding about the role as a center of the core, the hereditary information storage through their scientific outlook to expand.

The necessary equipment for training: computer technology, proektor, posters and slides.

Trainingcontent: the night of the core structure of the cell that is associated with the metabolic processes in different periods of life. Changing the core structure during ontogenez cells, especially the cells of these things and preparing to be when arising as a result of external influences of various. ,

Sitoplazma is much darker than the nucleus of plant cells. In general konsistensiyasi inside the core (composition) balzak, glycerin close by. The core of the plant is so dense that have konsistensiyasi but some of them can be cut into pieces, while some will be without half the liquid. It is able to change the shape of the core features. Sometimes ipsimon will take the form of changing the shape of the core. In exactly the same form the core of which is formed by way of kurtaklanib zamburug yeast cell to the new cell is moved.

The structure of the core

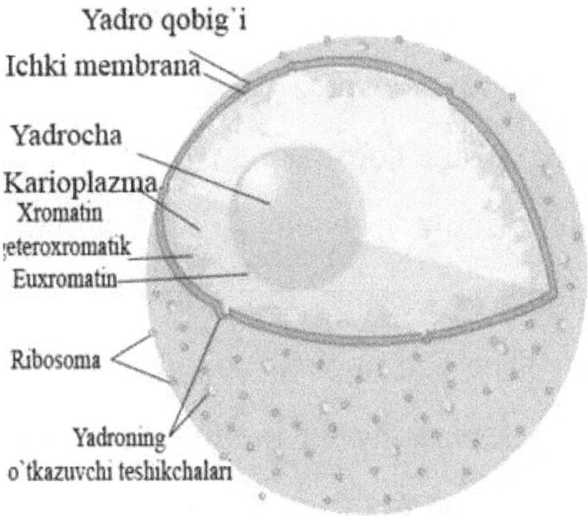

the main components of the core protein, nuklein acids, lipids, enzymes and mineral salts are. The core consists of the composition of simple and complex proteins. Giston from simple protein and globulin occurs. In addition to the structure of complex proteins aminoguruhdan again nuklein acids, carbohydrate occurs in the group (nukleoproteidlar, glikoproteidlar). Join with lipoproteidlar view tab in the lipid drop or proteidlar occurs. The amount of protein varies. They are the core of the dry weight of 10-20%

make up for it. Protein.synthesis of the active period is interfaza. Nuklein of two types of acid: dna and rna occurs. The main chemical component of the core dna, a part of chromosome DNA transmits genetic information from generation to generation; kodlaydi protein synthesis. The cell nucleus contains the dna from michelle f. separating for the first time in the year 1869. In addition to the dna in cells from the same core 3: information, at ribosoma and rna transport. Type in the cell nucleus giston more in the structure of proteins, the type of salt forms of the compounds with dna.

8.1-picture. The core of the structure.

So nogiston along with type of residual proteins. They diluted the salt does not dissolve in liquid. The same enzymes in the core ATV-bereavement, glikolitik there are enzymes, but enzymes are not oxidation. And by protein and lipids in the core network lipoproteidlar liponukleoproteidlar gistokimyoviy and biochemical methods, which had been found. They are the core of the dry weight of 10-20% make up for it.

In the core, calcium, magnesium, sodium, phosphorus, iron, zinc, copper, cobalt and other elem agent. xnts are also found.

Sitoplazma rna polymer possessing high conductivity of the crust from the core the core pass through modern information on hereditary information is of particular importance. If this hole is not the limit for ion tiny molecules on the one hand, on the second hand, a large rna molecules to pass ensures that informative sitoplazma. Sitoplazma from providing energy to the core and the nuclear large molecules that should be in sitoplazma sintezlanuvchi mononukleotid trifosfatning will take.

Purin amino acids, atp, active transport and by way of to the core of pirimidin passes. Sometimes the breakup of the substance can pass from the core the core is the idea that there sitoplazma. in turn the core in the shell] that appear from the same substance sitoplazma fagotsitoz like the cover.

The net yield is involved in the idea that there are sitoplazmatik the core in the shell. Profaza lace is combined with the shell in the core fragmentatsiyaga endoplamatik are structured. While the core element is formed from endoplazmatik telofazada shell from the back of the net. Thus, the core of the shell, the outer membrane, inner membrane, the cavity and core to ularorasidagi perinuklear openings.

Active surface which is open to the internet (site) is "locked" and will remain part of the same hereditary information from give. Thisin turn places the z chromosome in a cell varies depending on the position and possessing functional geteroxromatin euxromatin. The core of the activity of the cells of the rapid cycle will occur with some of geteroxromatinlarining euxromatinga some matters. Such xromatin geteroxromatindir optional. While geteroxromatin is Euxromatinlashmaydigan xromatin konstitutiv. Suppression of cell activity reduces the core of xromatin euxromatin takes place, that is sterilized to DNA euxromatin c, geteroxromatinga will go into.

Out of work: the theoretical part of the lesson, students are familiar with. Yadronong given in the picture composition, its components carefully they will do.

Constant location in its core by means of appropriate agreements drug through a microscope ko'ganingizda ribosoma attention. Give the importance of means of appropriate agreements and euxromatin geteroxromatinlar. The external and internal structure of the core on a sheet, 've drawn the picture above.

Control questions and assignments

1. Core functions in the cell, how?
2. Are there any parts in the core?
3. Ribosoma in the core occurs in which types?
4. The external and internal structure of the core on a sheet, 've drawn the picture above.

9-LABORATORY LESSONS

CHROMOSOME COMPOSITION AND STRUCTURE

Lesson aim: students of the chromosome structure and its components, give understanding about the role of chromosomes in cell life activity. Chromosome students and the types of its parts, through scientific understanding about the role of hereditary information storage center to give as expand their outlook.

The necessary equipment for training: computer technology, proektor, posters and slides.

Training content: the active surface, which is open to the internet (site) is "locked" and will remain part of the same hereditary information from give. Thisin turn places the z chromosome in a cell varies depending on the position and possessing functional geteroxromatin euxromatin. The core of the activity of the cells of the rapid cycle will occur with some of geteroxromatinlarining euxromatinga some matters. Such xromatin geteroxromatindir optional. While geteroxromatin is Euxromatinlashmaydigan xromatin konstitutiv. Suppression of cell activity reduces the core of xromatin euxromatin takes place, that is sterilized to DNA euxromatin c, geteroxromatinga will go into.

The chromosome structures with the beginning of the division of genetic factors Interfaza cases forms. Be completely metafaza of chromosomes are formed. They sentromerning in the form of chromosomes (any primary‘) according to the location of the three is the same: metasentrik, and submetasentrik akrotsentrik.

Metasentrik chromosome chromosome is located in the middle of sentromera xromrosomalar yelkali in particular for its equal.

Submetasentrik sentromera joylashmaydi in the middle of chromosome-chromosome, therefore the length of the chromosome yelkasi will be different.

The last of sentromera akrotsentrik chromosome chromosome (telomera) the part located close to chromosome g yelkasi one very long second while yelkasi will be very brief. Therefore, such a chromosome will be in the form of tayoqchasimon.

Any primary or Sentromerag' chromosomes during the division of cells to the spread of the pole provides. The chromosomes are pulled to the poles are combined and this axromatik ipchalar sentromeraga. Burama Sentromada stretched DNA of the chainqof chromosome-specific dna was roq sentromerada than other areas since the edge of theq chromosome painting and painted part with when it stays in the microscope without sentromera can be clearly seen. Sentromerasidan separated chromosomes reach the pole of the cell without in the next section is going to lose. Usually, a single chromosome is one sentromera. Many of sentromerali worm and insect chromosomes but some can be without.

Any primary chromosomeg‘ (sentromera) except from any secondary axromatik mix is combined. Therefore, it provides the direction of the chromosome to the pole. Any secondaryg‘yadrocha participates in some form and, therefore, referred to yadrocha ensure full compliance. Secondary yadrocha in the garden, and r-rna synthesis and the genes that will be located in managing reached its

Some secondary chromosome any chromosome is located near telomerasiga. Such a chromosome in any secondaryg‘dna in any secondary packaging was much the length of the chain sinceg‘from the next part, i.e. far away from telomerasi have a piece of chromosome settles, satellite builds. This part stands out with a strip adjacent satellite to satellite chromosome. People chromosomes among comrades also. For example, there are some people in chromosome kariotipidagi comrades.

Telomera - chromosome is the last part of chromosomes ensures the integrity and independence.

Pluck the parts of chromosomes can be easily combined with each other. But one of telomera kismi-never one does not merge with.

On the length of the chromosome inherited from the aspect of its activity is not the same. Painted with special paints chromosome when some parts of her painted dark and hungry while the other parts are painted, i.e. geteroxmatin euxromatin and builds.

The length of chromosomes 0,2-5,0 mkm, width 0.2-3,0 mkm can be. Some of the largest and hashorotlar amfibiyalar chromosomes,chromosomes, while fungi and suvo'tlar is tiny. Mkm chromosome is equal to the size of 1-10 people. The number and size of chromosomes in the organism incoming type should always be the same, always the same but it doesn't. The chromosome in the cells-cells with the same set of chromosomes is called.

Of chromosomes in the diploid somatic cells (2), while in the cells reach sexual gaploid (p) is in the package. 46 or 23 pairs in diploid cells of people (2), 8 or 4 pashshasi to drozofilla fruit in pairs.

The development of chromosome number in many of them the competence of the body-is not related to disruption. Many number of chromosomes that body (qisqichbaqasi the river, carp fish and others), less xromosomali to the body (man, monkey and etc) than can be configured very simply.

Profaza chromosome in the period gradually increases the size yo'g'onlashib will go. Metafaza later, will have the exact same shape. Therefore, the structure of the chromosome are usually studied in metafaza. Telofazaga later, ingichkalashib it again, uzunlashadi. Chromosomes are made of dna and protein complex is DNPdan.

The period in which the chromosomes of the cell matter eshilib buraluvchan, spiralsimon dezoksiribonukleoproteid is ipidan. The synthesis of two lengthwise and then gone from the period are equal to each other xromsomada the same part, i.e. xromat is formed. This xromatidalarning each dezoksiribonukleoproteid ipidan or xromoto occur.

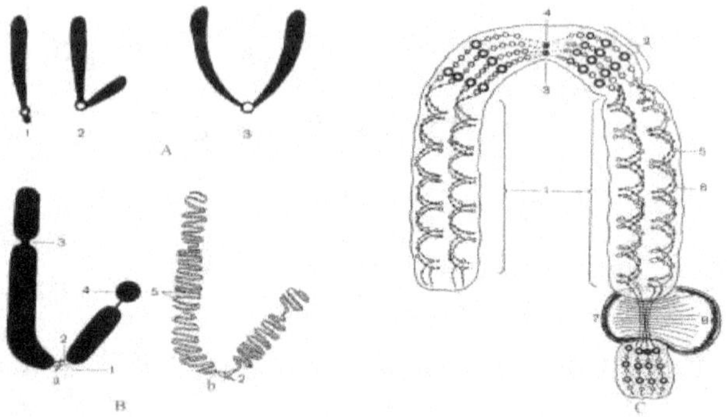

24- rasm. Xromosomaning tuzilishi. A- xromosoma xillari: 1- akrotsentrik; 2- submetatsentrik; 3- metatsentrik. B- xromosomaninituzilish sxemasi: a- tashqi ko'rinishi; b- ichki tuzilishi: 1- birlamchi belbog'; 2- sentromera; 3- ikkilamchi belbog'; 4- yo'ldosh; 5- xromonema. S- Xromosomaning ultramikroskomik tuzilish sxemasi: 1- euxromatin; 2- geteroxromatin; 3- birlamchi belbog'; 4- sentromera; 5- xromatida; 6- xromonema; 7- ikkilamchi belbog'; 8- yadrocha.

Of chromosome is generally from 20 to 200 pm which are composed of dna from xromofibrillalardan is very thin. Spirallashib chromosomes during cell division

While it can be interfaza ingichkalashib. Chromosome painting is called hromomeralar to the good part. Electronic Xromatin is seen in the microscope when its structure seems thin, that is can be three different xromatin fibrillarining yo'g'onligi: 250 a, 100 A, A. the third kind is considered fibrillalar intraoperative genetic 30-50 fibrillalar very active. As it is known, the diameter of a dna chain qo'sh 20, while the third kind in diameter 30-50 fibrillaning A. Therefore, the diameter of the third kind fibrillalarning protein (giston and gistonsiz) molecules at the expense of enlargement. 100 in a second fibrillalar the same diameter, different diameter of 30-50 a in the first fibrillalarning spirallashishidan, packaging is formed from. While the first kind, which is fibrillalar fibrillalarning spirallashishidan diameter 250 for the third time should be formed. Metafaza chromosome can be spirallashgan fibrillalar during the period in the third level. Spirallashgan these threads merged by mutual an electronic image which can be seen in the microscope when they are out of the chromosome.

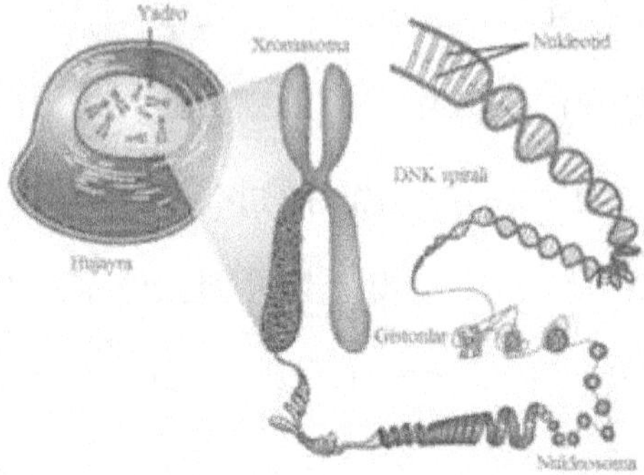

25- rasm. Xromosomaning tarkibiy qismlari.

In the structure having a molecular weight of 1000-2000 Dezoknukleoproteid strip (N1 N2A, N3V, N3, N4) gistonli in proteins occurs. While gistonsiz oksil is very poor, and they mostly repeat several tir xromatin ipchalar structure of enzymes and proteins, which consists of a collection of gistonli nukleosomalarga wrapped. Nukleosoma one of 4 different proteins (N2A, N2V, N3,N4) is formed mainly at the expense of two. The interaction of these proteins birlashgach, cylindrical sight similar to this will generate. Nukleosomaning active part two is one "core", the second is the "connecting" part is called.

“Connecting” part nukleosomalarni are tied with each other mutually. Nukleosomaning a-N1 gistonli proteins provides integrity and durability. Kalinligi of 1.5 nm of the dna spiral strip nukleosomaga head. The diameter of the association which is to be nukleosomadan dna and is equal to 10-13 nm.

20-25 nm in diameter from the combination of dna and protein strip ip spirallanishi more yield. Metafaza in ipni in having such a diameter can be seen using a microscope electronic interfaza. Again this is in the form of chromosomes in ipni spirallashishi as a result of his metafaza. The dna of the strip is reduced to 6 times its length as a result of nukleosomaga to be surrounded as a result of hereditary factors more unified is the convenience of the location in the chromosome.

Some of the chromosome number of the organism.

Chuchuk suv gidrasi	32	Meva pashshasi	8
Planariya	16	Uy pashshasi	12
Yomg'ir chuvalchangi	36	Sazan	104
Chig'anoqli bog' mollyuskasi	24,48	Olabug'a	28
Ot askaridasi	2,4	Triton	24
Daryo qisqichbaqasi	116 atrofida	Ko'l bakasi	24
It kanasi	28	Tez kaltakesak	38
O'rta Osiyo chigirtkasi	23	Kryakva o'rdagi	80
Suvarak	28	Kabutar	80
Bosh biti	12	Uy tovuklari	78
Shaftoli biti	12	Kuyon	44
Karam kapalagi	30	Echki	60
Uy sichqoni	40	Ko'y	54
Qunduz	30	Yevvoyi cho'chqa	40
Kalamush	42	Eshak	66
It	78	Prjevalskiy oti	66
Tulki	38	Ot	64
Mushuk	38	Makaka rezus maymuni	42
Qoramol	60		
Asalari	16,32	Shimpanze	48
Oddiy chivin	6	Odam	46

Independent test to complete the instructions:

1. How structured the nuclear membrane?

A. Qo'sh floor ; there ribosoma in the outer membrane, inner membrane smooth

B. Qo'sh floor: there are ribosoma in the inner membrane,the outer side is smooth

C. net Endoplazmatik with the participation of adjacent kanalli

With the floor wrapped in a membrane D.

2.Occurs no matter how the structure of the core juice

A. enzymes, amino acids

B. different proteins (including enzymes), free nucleotides, and amino acids, which is associated with the core and from the core activities of life xromatin sitoplazma out which products to

C. lipid,protein.carbohydrate

D. protein,fat,nukleoprotein.aminoklslotalar.

Savo and assignments

1. I've mitoz the structure of chromosome.
2. Xromatin structure
3. Xromatin proteins
4. The structure of the chromosome level
5. Xromosomaning the fine structure and its formation

10-LABORATORY LESSONS
MITOZ PROCESS

Hobbiesto order: mitoz mitoz phase of the study and its importance.

The necessary equipment for training: computer technology, proektor, posters, tablitsalar and slides

Training content: the process is in the cell on the basis of certain qonuniyat go to them to come in the series and can be mitoz interfaza. Some populations of cells will be constantly (kambial zone cells). Be the preparation time (interfaza) and be joined mitoz mitoz cycle is called.

Interfaza begin the formation of the structure and within the cells during the period of sharp growth. To this period $\mathbf{G_1}$-synthesis of the period before it is called. During this period of intensive biochemical characterized by protein and rna synthesis, which is the time of the cell generating 30-40% for accounts.

S during the period of which have long formed the core of the bad paint xromatin confused and mutually accept (except if geteroxromatin). Then I will take you to the period of dna synthesis. This synthetic period, during this period of dna synthesis in the core kuzitiladi. Time generating 30-50% of the nitrogen in this period accounted for a part of the basis of the dna spesifik xromatin timi's core. Xromasoma as a result of the synthetic period, namely the generation of cells of the material that is two times the increase in the period after s.

G_2 -mitoz before the period, come prepared to be characterized by the cell. This period of time generating 10-20% for accounts. G2-period, after generating the time of 5-10% accounted for the m - mitoz is the start of the period.

Mitoz is the difference in phase 4 of the process at:

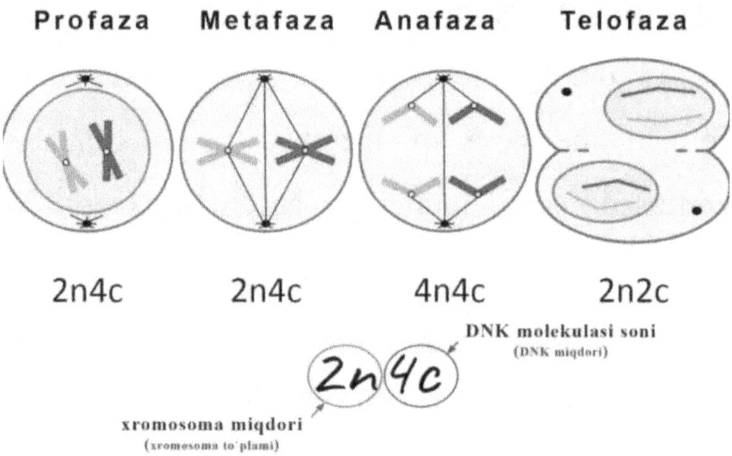

10.1-picture. Mitoz process.

Procondensation of the chromosomes and the formation of an apparatus mitoz phase is observed. Xromoyo'g'onlashib will increases the size of the soma. Profaza xromotodlarning formed around this event during the period not to become one of the latter, but each one of himself, a spiral creates. In the next phase of separated mitoz therefore they will light up. Profaza xromotidlardan was founded at the end of the chromosome pair. Along with swelling and xromasoma yo'g'onlashib be called sentromeralar known xromatidlar is combined with. At the end of the chromosome Profaza bo'linayotgan ekvatorial settles on the surface of the core, in the form of dukchi to be started. State unitary enterprise from ipchalar type two-pole pole xromasoma of combining central and combining with the proverbial proverbial ipchalar sentromerlari from the chromosome was founded. Mitoz an electronic apparatus from the tube walls of the dense mikroskopiya ipchalar had found that shows up. Their diameter is 20 nm, the wall thickness of 4-5 nm.

Dukchi sentriolalar displaces the opposite pole of the core depending on sentriolalar between animals. Dukchi size increases at this time, the core xarakterliki the crust is melted. Electron microscopic observations in the period mitoz not to lose the core of the crust slices, but sitoplazmatik membrane showed that the net has become. Mitoz endoplazmatik net core is formed from the membrane re-structured at the end of the shell.

Metafaza ekvatorial completely formed in the surface will be located in the chromosome. Chromosome the chromosome of an apparatus that may act depending on chromosomes dukkam senromerlarining mitoz ends with threads of the merger (the star of the plate or ekvatorial motherhood).

Mitakinez (chromosome dukkam actions) are relatively perpendicular to the goverment's unitary plant ipchalar as a result of the chromosome lies in the number of chromosomes such their location, and will help to determine great shape. The number of chromosomes in each type of creature known to exist. Each of the two copies of the same chromosome in the same

phase-tah xromat after finding the subscriber is seen.

Anafaza-xromatidalarning begins from the chromosome are separated from each other. At this time, the girl that form the chromosome each chromosome (xromat) I will try depending on the opposite pole. In this way “the girl's a star” is in the form of. Sinxron in the movement of chromosomes on the same night. This mechanism of action is still no'malum.

Telofaza-mitoz the last period. Its beginning, the goverment's unitary plant chromosome /cell/ will come to the opposite pole. Profaza telofaza as if it is the opposite of all the processes in the reverse order goes. State unitary enterprise lose buralgan the chromosome, spreading uzunlashadi, the core of the girl re-restored yadrocha kobig'i and core is formed. Mitoz will take place in the cells of the body and broken down of the hardware (or sitotomiya sitokinez). Thetrack interfaza will have a specific structure to the cells in the nucleus of the cells. Sitotomiya mechanism explored enough yet.

Out of work: the theoretical part of the lesson, students are familiar with. Mitoz mitoz video training process even more deeply learn and reflected again through the process step-by-step photos to draw pictures of the trail.

1-assignments. The stages of the process, respectively, which reflect the number of pictures Mitoz write to the table.

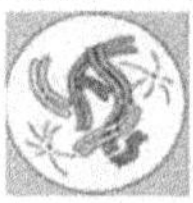	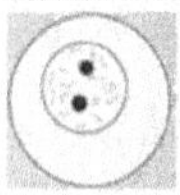	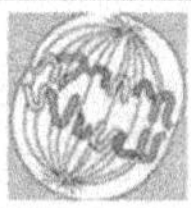	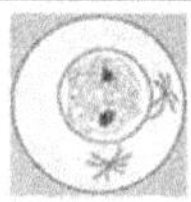
1	2	3	4
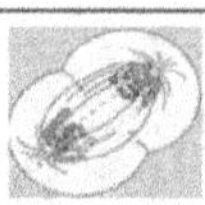	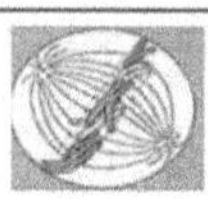	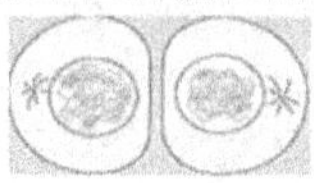	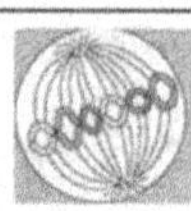
5	6	7	8

Interfaza –	Profaza –	Metafaza –	Anafaza –	Telofaza –

The question of control

1. Cells what is a life cycle?

2. Mitoz cycle what is it?
3. Interfaza of the period.
4. Profaza the processes that occur in life.
5. How metafaza processes in the cells during the period happens?
6. Anafaza processes that go in.
7. Telofazada chromosome changes.
8. Mitoz process modeling.

11-LABORATORY LESSONS
MEYOZ PROCESS. PROCESS MODELING
MEYOZ

Hobbiesto order: Mostudy of the phase of the bit.

The necessary equipment for training: Meyoz reflected tablitsalar process, computer technology, proektor, posters and slides.

General concept: Meyoz – sexual in a way that increase observed in plants, and the core of utis gaploid xromosomali condition ensures that diploid status. The method of closed plants flower and seeded urug'kurtagi changdonida this division is realized. "Meyoz" terminology of the German "meyoz the word" is derived from "reduce" means. The reason that it had reduced the number of chromosomes in this section, "reduktsion" to be called.

Meyoz consists of 2 stages:

1)is formed from two diploid somatic cells sex cells xromosomali gaploid xromosomali.

2) mitoz (similar to ekvatsion)at each of two similar sexual cells gaploid xromosomali sex cells are formed. Them later (or as a result of micro makrogametogenez) gameta comes in the form of male or females.

Meyoz every phase of phase consists of 4 units: profaza, metafaza, and anafaza telofaza.

Profaza to change depending on the internal structure of the core stage 1 stage 5 my youngest is divided into:

1) leptonema;

2) zigonema;

3) paxinema;

4) diplonema;

5) diakinez.

Leptonemada tursimon ipsimon core structure and the diploid number.

Zigonemada xromatin threads lengthwise and pull one of each pair from the top side and gives away kon'yugatsiya united.

Paxinemada gomologik 4 units of chromosome pairs xromat is to be united, and this condition is called tetrada.

Diplonema zigonemaning the opposite, gomologik from the top side of the chromosome, of the form x-shaped and separated from each other is formed. This condition is called xiazma.

Diakenezda xromatidlar yo'g'onlashib will most driving.

Metafaza 1 pair of chromosomes at the equator line at gomologik places across yadrocha peel and core is dissolved.

Anafaza 1 chromosome pair at gomologik mutual divorce started. This is referred to as in dia. Each pair are separated one from each chromosome to the poles. Therefore, the harvest of the cells of the body equal to half of the sex cells will pass.

1 Telofaza yadrocha bark and core loss at axromatik threads is formed. The first stage of meyoz the same ends.

The chromosome number from diploid cells in the first phase of meyoz xromosomali gaploid which is a quad-core dual-core cell is formed (dia are). While in stage 2 of meyoz gaploid package which is able to dual-core from the cell, four quad-core (tetrada) appear in the cells. Meyoz of the period between the stage and reduktsion ekvatsion interkinez is called.

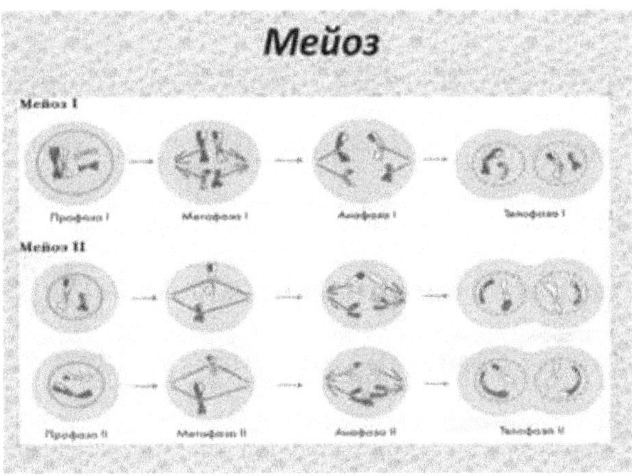

11.1-picture. Meyoz process

Mainly sexual and jinssiz method is increased in the body. Fertilization through sexual reproduction is realized. While jinssiz reproduction, spores (fungi) and vegetative method is realized.

Increased in the vegetative method (when they tuganaklar, onions and h.k.) hereditary does not change the state of plants. Therefore, in practice, since this method is widely used. For example, the rapid increase in uniquely varieties, varieties of fruit trees, vine, berries, potatoes, sarimsoqpiyoz vegetative organs is carried out by breeding crops also like. In addition, the effect of geterozis saved by breeding with the same method also can include.

Sexual reproduction male and female reproductive cells of the body – the form of adding gameta, that is, formed from the fertilized from zigota.

Zigota – the fertilized egg cell, the first cell of a new generation is increased by way of mitoz and will become the new body.

Out of work: the theoretical part of the lesson, students are familiar with. Tablitsa or video through process and learn the lessons again even deeper meyoz Meyoz reflected the process step-by-step photos to draw pictures of the trail.

The question of control

1. I've Meyoz the meaning of the word
2. List the stages of the process Meyoz
3. The biological significance of meyoz
4. Meyoz process modeling.

12- LABORATORY LESSONS

THE STUDY OF THE SIMILARITIES AND DIFFERENCES OF PLANT AND ANIMAL CELLS

Purpose of training: the structure of plant and animal cells, they have similarities and differences study.

Necessary materials and equipment: Microscopes, parts and window yopqich far priproval needle, scalpel, fuksin oil paint, oil immersion, pipetka, an alcohol lamp, 96% alcohol li, cotton, fork, ripe tomatoes, briar, pepper, fruit, animal, carpet runner, the hair fiber. constant of the prepared drugs of plant and animal cells, the cell on the composition of tables.

Theoretical concepts: Animal cells, plant cells compared to vary with the following features:

1) cells have a high level of specialization, that is, the second function can fulfill the demands of the different cells of the same cell;

2) come out from the function of the cell b xilmaxil the form o ‘lish; and

3) special form orgonoidlarni;

4) the formation of blastometrlar.

The main features of the plant cell are the following:

1) each cell of the external base layer — shell cell ‘accounted for its existence;

2) be a system of permanent vakuol;

3) organella protoplastd m axsus — plastida availability;

4) ergastik (nutrients, harmful products), the accumulation of substances.

5) in the case of the living cell specialization and secondary embrional the back o ‘o zgarib ‘teeth;

6) kariokinezda sentriolaning sitokinezda fragmoplastlarning be formed.

Assignments: 1. Study the structure of plant cells. 2. Study the structure of animal cells.

Out of work: ripe tomatoes, pepper and slices of fruit or briar who was dropping the scalpel out of the water using products priproval nina is put window, window covering, then the items great while initially a microscope of small objects is observed.

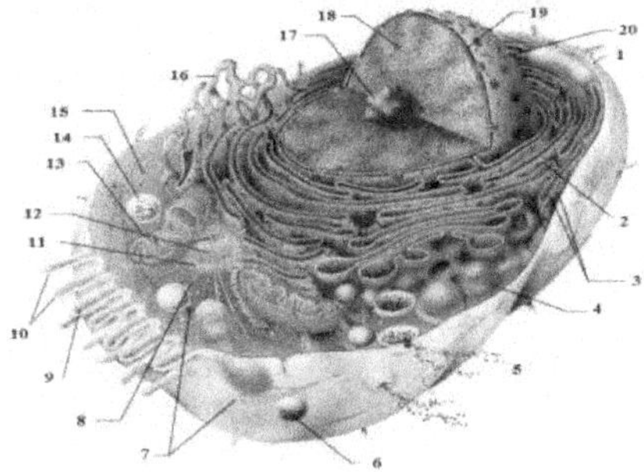

4–rasm. Hujayralarning ultramikroskopik tuzilishi (sxema).

1 – hujayra qobig'i (sitolemma); 2– donador endoplazmatik to'r; 3– ribosoma; 4–Golji apparati; 5– sekret ajratma; 6–peroksisoma; 7– oraliq filomentlar; 8– mikronaychalari; 9– mikrofilamentlar; 10– mikrovorsinkalar; 11– sentrosoma; 12– sentriol (hujayra markazi) 3– mitoxondriya; 14– lizosoma; 15– gialoplazma; 16– silliq endoplazmatik to'r; 17– yadrocha; 18– xromatin; 19– yadro qobig'i; 20– yadro.

Po'st consi ts of thin circular cell in the fact that his xloroplast, xromoplast, and other leykoplast of organoid seems to be clear.

Animal carpet runner lupa hair fiber and examined under a microscope, the structure of the study and draw a picture of them.

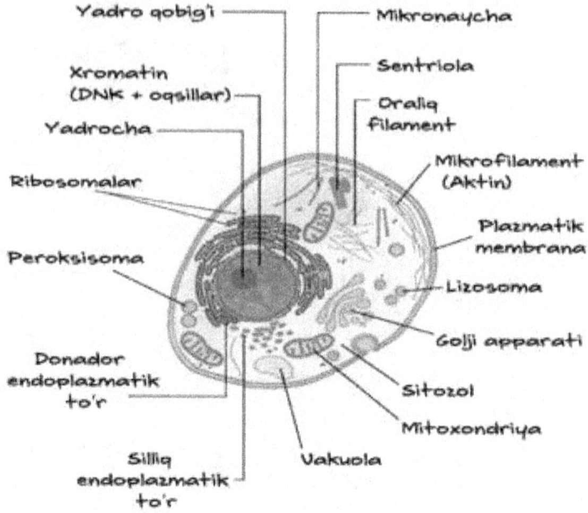

12.2-picture. The structure of animal cells.

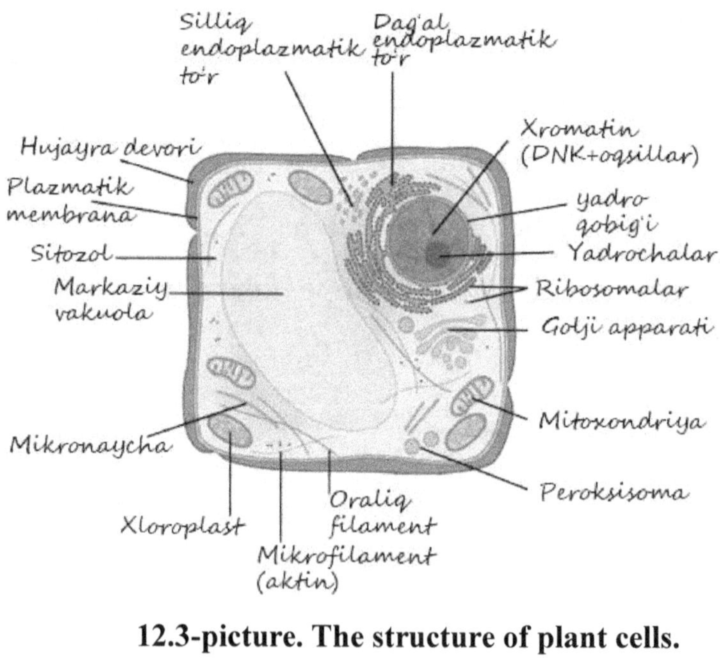

12.3-picture. The structure of plant cells.

Write the parts of the cell, respectively, in the following picture.

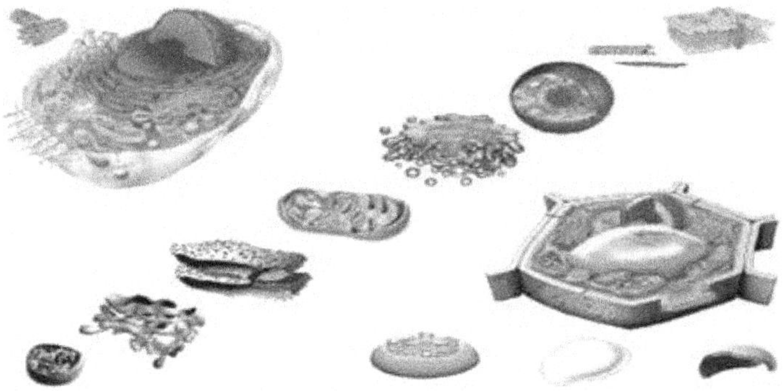

Control questions and assignments

1. I've the structure of plant cells.
2. What the difference consists of animal and plant cells.
3. Let us explain the structure and function Xromoplastning.
4. The bark of the structure of the cell I have.
5. Organellalari cells: mitoxondriya, Goldji apparatus endoplazmatik lace, ribosoma, membrane, plastida, the xloroplast, leykoplast,

xromoplast fill your table with the proper understanding and proteins.

6. 've drawn the picture of the animal and plant cells.

13- LABORATORY LESSONS

ONE-STOREY TISSUE EPITELIY

Mashg'lulotining purpose: one-storey structure kubsimon epiteliy, briefly in her study of the method of preparation of the drug. One-storey structure will have understanding about kubsimon epiteliy they will comment on.

The necessary equipment for training: thematic tablitsalar, microscope, drugs constantly, slides, cards created.

Theoretical concepts:

One-story, one lane epiteliy dm-mezoteliy

A lane epiteliy dm: cystic lung, the pleura, the wall of the heart the surface of the bag, gavin bora charvi wall and cavity cover. Also the liver, spleen and ovaries bora closed (covered) is.

The external and internal surface of the body along with trophic mezoteliy complete the task the cover and ensures the smooth surface of the form and structure of the active movement jaroxatlanishdan saves. If you tore out of the organs of connective tissue growth adjacent to it here and grow. (spa). This course pathology.

Kiprikli epiteliy dm (mezoteliy). This type of tubal epiteliy mainly occurs in the body of the animals. Dm cells forms kubsimon section and cylindrical, apical part is covered with kiprikchalar. M: to‘o garakg‘gauge (the mino to miksinalarda) cylindrical, amfibiyalar kubsimon in his ujayralar.

Epithelial - dm epiteliy muscles (mioepiteliy) Such epiteliy the kovakichlilarda occurs in the basal part of the cell is located miofibriallar. It is also said that the same mioepiteliy. Selomik animals (xalqa a) worms, clams (bo'g'imoyoqlilar, ninatanlilar)mezoteliy the surface of the secondary body cavity is covered.

Out of work: one-storey kubsimon the part of the drug under a microscope to see epitileyni buyragi kernels should be prepared from rabbits. Kubsimon epitiley deametrdagi yig'uv kanalcha small wall cover.

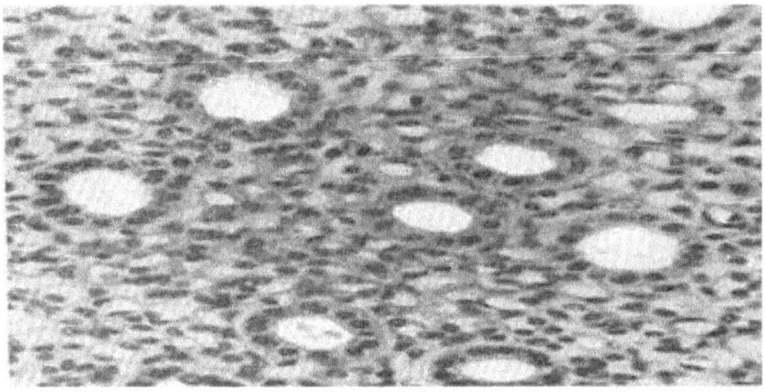

13.1-picture. A tiny rabbit collector channel buyragi kubsimon of epiteliy

Preparatda of almost the same diameter to afford kanalcha is removed. Kanalcha equal to the width of the edge of the wall, i.e. in the form of cells kubsimon epitiley will cover. Sitoplazma apical part of the cells to'qroq a bit, while the other part is painted a color to a light pink color, and dark purple in color, while the core of looks.

When you see the great object of the microscope the cells with basal membrane put limits can be clearly seen. Soft to the cells in the connective tissue around the core of urine yig'uv kanalcha painted a dark purple color. Here also cross-cuts in the tiny vessels occurs.

A dm-storey epiteliy. Charvi total drug prepared from whole colon (salt painted with silver nitrate). (Mezoteliy); finding small objects under a microscope a very thin cut of the drug drug mezoteliy place because here it seems clear cells are seen. Large objective under the border of the cell (1) is found, and studied the picture are drawn. Give importance to the shape of the cell.

To the core (2) detection, dual-core cell (3) and specify in the picture find.

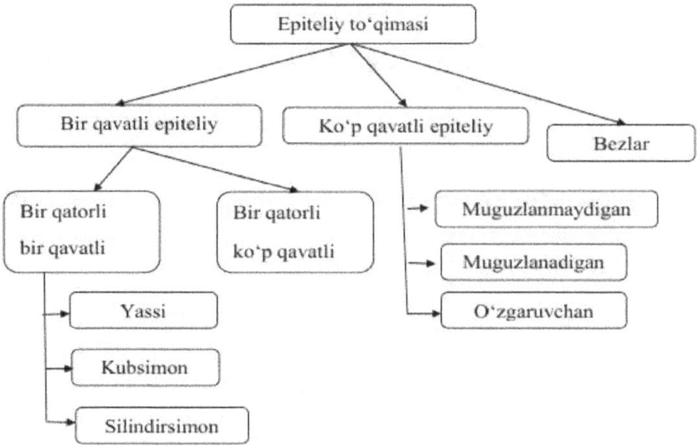

Questions and assignments

1. Which parts of the animal's body will appear in Kubsimon epiteley?
2. Buyragi looks in a microscope of any color in epiteliy kubsimon rabbit?
3. Epiteley any type of tissue is to be?
4. 've drawn on the photos of laboratory sessions.

14-LABORATORY LESSONS

MULTI-STOREY TISSUE EPITELIY

Mashg'lulotining purpose: lane many a case-kiprikli results epiteliy structure, briefly in her study of the method of preparation of the drug. Laboratory mshg'uloti as a result, many students in lane a case-kiprikli epiteliy they will comment on results about the structure of understanding.

The necessary equipment for training: thematic tablitsalar, microscope, drugs constantly, slides, cards created.

Theoretical concepts:

Multi-storey epiteliy

Multi-storey floor consists of multiple epiteliy if it is located on one of the floors. The floor of each cell are different from each other according to the structure and function fulfilled. Multi-storey epiteliy the body of vertebrate animals, the most part is covered. In particular: the skin, ogiz cavity, the esophagus, the veil of the eye, the internal surface of the sexual organs of women, urine qopi surface is covered. They are microscopic different composition than 3: muguzlanmaydigan, muguzlanadigan and changing.

Muguzlanmaydigan multi-storey flat epiteliy people and animals ogiz cavity, esophagus, eye spots occurs. There is not Muguz the floor.

Muguzlanadigan multi-storey flat epiteliy. The skin of humans and animals: the skin consists of two parts. 1. The epidermis of 2. Dermal or skin chin-dermidi to 4-5 from the floor. The heel and kaftda floor 5, 4 in the floor, the rest, i.e. in the floor will not be all shiny.

1.The increase of the basal cells in the form of floor or floor tsilinrsimon be, and increased stand features. 2.The cells of the barbed floor (a few layers), sometimes split increased.

3. Structured floor

4. Shiny floor

5. Muguzlangan floor

6. Basal curtains

7. True skin

Variable (was proverbial) epiteliy_always stick tension and relax the body functions according to these fulfilled the inner surface of the stand is covered. These jomi to the kidney, urine and body fluid when filled with qopi is the width of the cell if it goes out of the liquid returns back to the original version.

Sekret epiteliy changing some cells from the surface of cells and for the production of urine zax keep re-absorbed would not let urine.

Order of work: Many of the internal surface of the respiratory tract epiteliy lane kiprikli cylindrical cover. See small objects initially focus of the drug, kekirdak (trachea) which cover the inner surface of large objects after finding epiteliy existence is held.

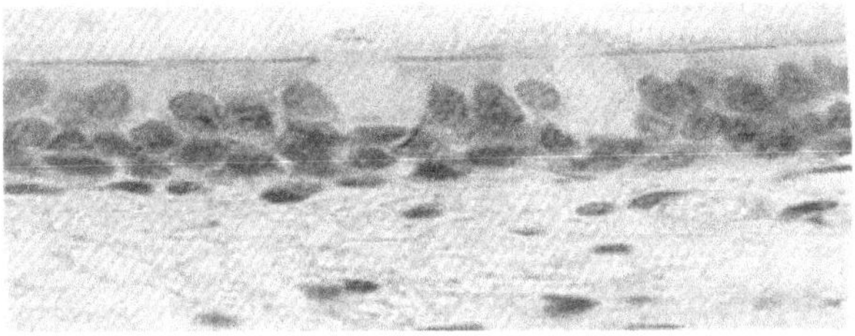

14.1-picture. A lot of muscle in the trachea lane a case-epiteliy results

Many xilpillovchi lane kiprikli epiteliy a few different cells. The length of the roll and the short space consists of cells. Among them qadahsimon occurs in many cells. The shape and length of all of these in spite of being different approach to the basal membrane touch.

A case-kiprikli epiteliy results of the edge length, has a cylindrical shape. The basal part of the cell membrane to touch the proverbial small, i.e. the expansion of the apical part of the tissue surface to high stands out. Located on the apical membrane in the part we will see dense lashes. The space length of each cell in a different form, with the expansion part is to touch the basement membrane. The upper part of the tissue surface to ingichkalashib not out. Sitoplazma is located in the center of the core of the cell. The expansion will also touch the membrane with the basal part of the cells of the small space, but a large space from the edge in terms of the cell is much lower in the basal part of the cell nucleus. Kiprikchalar the space in both cells are not, they rise to the surface of the tissue, despite the fact that cells are located among kiprikli epitiliy. Three cells in the core of many tissue under the microscope being reinforced by three different lane, it looks like.

The structure of the tissue and gland cells occurs in a cell except for the space and cylindrical qadahsimon. Out of the surface of the tissue product of the gland, and is sent out with keeping dust from entering the air will remain.

The changing of the bladder multi-storey epiteliy of.

Focus on small objects in tissue birikturuvchi (2) layer, which lay epiteliy (1) find.

Pay attention to large objects form the floor epiteliy few number of nuclear focus. In basal membrane (3) which lay kubsimon (4) to examine and take noksimon certain cells. While on this hujayralaming, flat cells (5) is located. Sitoplazma cells (6) and the core

(7) to identify.

To complete the task independently

1. Cylindrical lane kiprikli many epiteliy study the structure of the tissue.
2. Many qanarrowcylindrical li kiprikli epiteliy location and importance in the body of the analysis.
3. Determine the apical and basal part of the essence.
4. Draw pictures on laboratory sessions.
5. Epiteliy determine tissue contrast from other features.

15-LABORATORY LESSONS

LEARN THE STRUCTURE OF THE GLAND

The purpose of training: the types of glandular structure epiteleyning and learn.

Necessary materials and equipment: thematic tablitsalar, microscope, drugs constantly, slides, cards created.

Theoretical concepts: epiteliy Glandular - ekzo in the body - and the form of endocrine glands. Special material glands - sekret production. Sekret parchalovchi the various ingredients enzymes, or other substances can be mucous. They basically ekzokrin is produced in the thyroid gland. Endocrine glands-the world of special effects in executive, managing agents is the use of hormones in the various processes of life.

Epiteliy glandular cells of the gland - cells sekretor glandulositlardan - ekzokrinositlardan is. Glandulositlar special substances - the work of sekret*and lab members hypothyroidism builds. Ekzokrin two different glands and endocrine glands. We are here we are giving a general description ekzokrin gland(15.1-picture). Histology of the endocrine glands are studied in private.*

*Ekzokrin gland cell (qadahsimon cells) and hug a lot-jayra will be. Sekretor chiqaruv Ekzokrin stem consists of glands and the last. The glandular Ekzokrin*the classification of er:

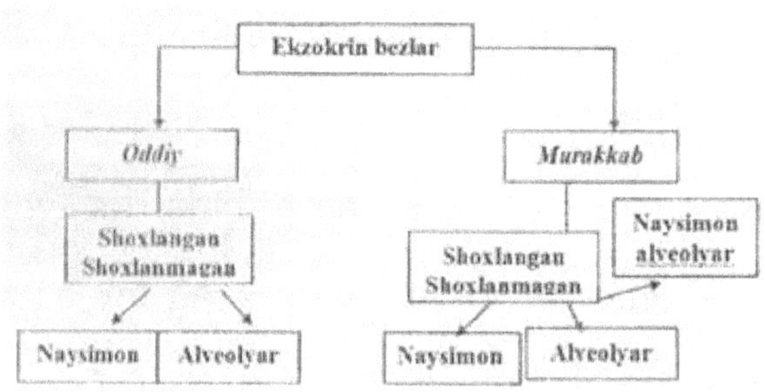

Ekzokrin the secretion of glands in the outer gland (endocrine glands of the inner sec-retsiya glands) is called. The product of the gland Ekzokrin - sekret chiqaruv through the stem to the external environment - the surface of the skin, the members poured into the cavity.

Simple stem shoxlanmagan chiqaruv in the thyroid gland, the gland complex, while in stem or in stem chiqaruv the last of the mixture and a few naysimon alveolar shoxlangan chiqaruv will be opened. Ektoderma will be the last of which is formed from the gland cells occurs in around mioepitelial. Oqsilli the last sections of the gland (serous), slime (mukoz), mixed (seromukoz) groups according to the type allocated to the use of sekret, the gland protein, mucous, fat, sweat gland is.

Sekretor sekret separation in cells from the cell (secretion) is the same as 4.

1. Merokrin - sitolemmasi this cell does not break.

2.Mikroapokrin cell apical sitolemmasida to break a small-s.

3.Makroapokrin - sitolemmasida apical cell disorders is large.

Golokrin - cells completely broken down (15.2-picture).

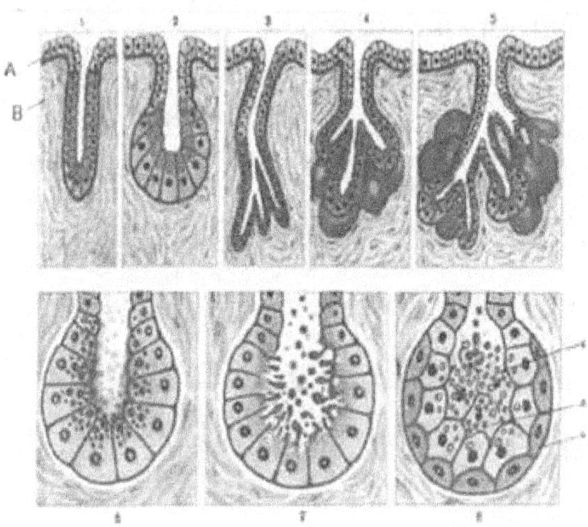

***15.1-15.2-pictures.* The secretion of the gland and its types.** A-glandular epiteliy B-connective tissue. 1-5-types of the gland; 6-merokrin; 7-apokrin; 8-golokrin secretion.

Lo gland endocrine gland ekzokrin know the difference from put-is rhodes. Special substances and the form of the endocrine system endocrine glands - hormones will work. Chiqaruv stem directly towards them, and does not have much more productive in the blood is poured into the lymph tissue. Along with nervous system function was the management of hormones. The endocrine glands are mainly endoderma mezenximadan and development.

Out of work: Drugs, elektronogrammalar, posters and learning scheme, draw the structure of the principles of epiteliy album.

I. a brief note of the drug.

1. Simple tarmoqlanmagan naysimon glands. Focus on small objects birikturuvchi the drug in the skin tissue (1) limited with the amount of toe‘-of the christian community, in the last part of the piece gland (2), was directed to the side of yom epiteliy chiqaruv (3) find.

Large objects focus in basal membrane (4) is located in the last part of kubsimon sekretor or cylindrical epithelial cells (5). find Kubsimon epiteliy (6) identify ways and chiqaruv covered with connective tissue. Multi-storey and skin muguzlanuvchi (7) epiteliy chiqaruv find the way within. Parmasimon give importance to the form of the yoi.

2. Simple naysimon the gastric gland of the bottom of the drug.

Focus on small objects of gastric mucous membranes (1). find Large objects cylindrical shaped gland epiteliy focus of the cover (2) study. Under it is a simple composition that has a glandular stem (3) to find. This gland is in the neck (4) body (5), the bottom (6) to find. The depth of the pancreatic gland stem (7) give the importance of opening. A floor made from the cells located in the basal membrane of the gland, despite a diversity of differently sized and painted

in the form of the cells occurs in both. These cells was different functions. Additional in the structure of the gland (8) key (9) and pariyetal cells (10) is the difference.

3. Tarmoqlangan alveolar gland complex. Salivary gland front of the ear. Objective structured under the capsule surrounding the gland small gland from the connective tissue (1), find the movement of the capsule gland located under slices. The cone-shaped epithelial cells sekretor focus on large objects from s (4) structured sekretor the last part (3). see The cells under mioepitelial cells (5). find Find ways chiqaruv formed from flat epithelial cells. You can also learn the structure of the gland in the scheme. Last sekretor between the parts of the cavity (8), which is slightly wider linear salivary bomib of the stem (8) to find. Ways of epithelial cells of the cylindrical wall (9) is formed. The basal part of these cells (10) lines. BoMakchalar between thin connective tissue layer (12) wrapped with pieces of-of-of the stem (13) to determine.

II. 1. Electronic mikrofotografiyalar:

1. Electronic mikrofotografiyasi Qadahsimon of the cell.
2. Kekirdak kiprikli of epiteliy.

Questions and assignments

1. Glandular epiteley of any type is to be?
2. Sekretor what is it?
3. Ekzokrin bring an example to the gland.
4. Bring to the example of the endocrine gland.
5. How bezib front of the ear, salivary gland example?
6. **I've been sekresiya into the specific answer:** 1) apokrin; 2) merokrin; 3)golokrin; 4) does not destroy the cells in merokrin sekresiya; 5) the secret ekzokrin gland into the blood passes.

7. **Find the fit issues**

1) Ektoderma a) the tip of the cell is broken;

2) Apokrin b) the epidermis;

3) Golokrin v) the fat gland;

4) epiteliy Dm g) in the stomach is bomib;

5) Sekretor cells d) mezoteliy.

List of used literature:

Rahbariy literature:

1.Mirziyoyev Sh.M. Critical analysis strictly order-discipline and personal responsibility – the daily rule of every business leader should be. The cabinet of ministers of the republic of uzbekistan the year of the end of 2016 and 2017. the president of the republic of uzbekistan, dedicated to the prospects of speech. // The word people newspaper. 2017. January 16, №11

2. Mirziyoyev Sh.M. We will build our great future together and our nation with courage and noble. "Uzbekistan", 2017.

3. Mirziyoyev Sh.M. To ensure you can maintain the rule of law and the interests of the people and the people faravonligi is the guarantee of the development of the country. "Uzbekistan", 2017

Basic literature:

1. Abdulov. I. A. Halbekova. H. i. cell biology. Textbooks, Tashkent,Donishmand Ziyo“ -2020.

2. Toshmanov N., R. Madatov, the development of biology. textbooks, Tashkent 2022 y.

3. Toshmanov N., the development of biology. textbooks, Tashkent 2018 y

4. Tuichiyev S. N. Toshmonov “Cytology, embryology, histology” textbook. Tashkent, 2005 y.

5. To'ychiev. S Toshmanov N., Fayzullaev S. “Cytology, embryology, histology” (study guide), Tashkent:, 2004 y.

6. Eshonqulov e. o., and n. K. Nishonboyev b. “Cell biology and development” (study guide), Tashkent, 2010. Electronic.

7. L Belousov.V. Osnovi obtshey embriologii. - Moscow: MGU, 2005.

8. A Dondua. K. Biology razvitiya. T. 1, 2. - Sp has.: Izda-where Spbgu, 2005.

9. B. Xoliqnazarov Induvidual the development of biology. Tashkent, 2006.

Additional literature:

1. Shodiev N. SH. Cytology, histology and embryology. "Labor."
–Tashkent, 2006. (corrected and filled 2-edition).
2. Ibragimov Sh.I. N. Yusupov Sh. A.. Daminov Cytology,
3. Histology and embryology. "Labor." – Tashkent, 1998.
4. E. Kodirov Histology. Labor. T.: 2012.Kuznesov S.L., Mushkambarov N.N., Goryachkina.V.L. Po histological atlas,

tsitologii I embriologii. 'Medisinskoe informativnoe agentstvo'. Moscow, 2002.

5. N. a. Manuilova the basics of histology and embryology. Tashkent, Teachers', 1970. 286 page.
6. K. i. Salixbaev the development of biology. Tashkent, ToshDU, 1992.
7. Vine May B. P. Obtshaya embryology / B. P. The vine may be. M. :Uzbekistan. branch., 1987.
8. Albert, S. B. Molekulyarnaya biology kletki. T. 1-3. - Moscow: Mir, 1994.
9. Almazov, *I. V.* Histological atlas I embriologii I po/. V. Almazov, L. S. Sutulov.M. : Medisina, 1978.
10. Volkov, O. V. Histology, cytology and embryology I: Atlas. / O. V. In Volkov, Yu. K. Eleskiy. M. : Medisina, 1996.

11. Golichenkov, *V. A.* Praktikum po embriologii / V. A. Golichenkov, M. L. In simeon.M. :Academy, 2004.
12. From general histology i. k. kodirov practical lessons. Methodical guide. Tashkent.1983 y.
13. V Eliseev.G., Afanasev Yu.I. Walk N.A. Histology. M."Medisina",1983
14. Not gilbert. F.,BarresiM.J.F. DevelopmentalBiology. 11th ed. - Sunderland, massachusetts, usa, 2016.940 p.
15. S In Aleksandrov.A. Bogolyubova. The molecularie osnovi I kletochnie in ontogenez. Saint-Petersburg. Izda-where.polytechnical. un-ta, 2011. -230 s.
16. Golichenkov, *V. A.*Embryology / V. A. Golichenkov, E.A.Ivanov, E.N.Nikeryasova.M. :Academy, 2004.

18. Column N.V., N Volkov.E. Vorobeva L.G. In ontogenez engine. Izda-where to Kharkiv. Un-ta –2015. - 220.s.

19. Ostroverxova G.P., Ostroverxovas. N.V. I razvitiya bespozvonochnix razmnojeniya biology. Tomsk. Izda. Dom Tomskogo gosudarstvennogo university, 2015. – 464 s.

20. Gilbert S. Biology razvitiya. M.: Mir, 2010. 840 s.

Internet sites:

1. http://php.med.unsw.edu.au/embryology
2. http://www.sdbonline.org
3. www.ziyonet.uz..
4. www.maik.ru.
5. www.libmmn.h.15.ru
6. http://elbrary.ru/projects/citation/citation_info.asp
7. twripx.com

www.ingramcontent.com/pod-product-compliance
Lightning Source LLC
Chambersburg PA
CBHW062141160726
48282CB00027B/891

* 9 7 8 9 3 6 9 0 8 8 5 6 0 *